Ketogenic Therapy fo

Transforming Fat into Energy

Note

Medicine is constantly changing. Standardized safety measures should always be adopted, and as new research and clinical experiences expand our knowledge, there may be a need to change or adapt the therapeutic protocol and the use of medicines. This book is aimed at the general public. Its content is intended for information purposes and may not be suitable for all readers. The contents of this book do not replace medical advice. Everyone should always see their doctor before making any health-related decisions. The publisher and the author do not assume any liability for any damage and/or injury to persons arising from this publication.

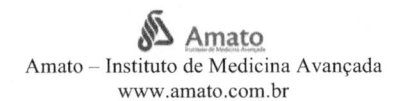

Ketogenic Therapy for Lipedema

Transforming Fat into Energy

Alexandre Campos Moraes Amato

Amato – Instituto de Medicina Avançada
www.amato.com.br

1st edition
São Paulo, SP
2023

Copyright © 2023 by Dr. Alexandre Campos Moraes Amato

All rights reserved.

No part of this publication may be reproduced, stored in a retrieval system, or transmitted in any form or by any means, electronic, mechanical, photocopying, recording, or otherwise, without the author's prior written permission. When not created by the author, the images were provided with permission.

First print:

ISBN: **9798869906304**
V 1.0

Amato – Instituto de Medicina Avançada
Av. Brasil 2283
São Paulo, SP, 01431-001
www.amato.com.br

Author, name
   Ketogenic Therapy for Lipedema – Transform Fat Into Energy / Author, Alexandre Campos Moraes Amato – São Paulo, SP, 2023. ISBN:
9798869906304

Appendices
Includes table of contents

Presentation

Losing weight, healthily getting more energy, improving your health, reducing inflammation, and treating various diseases, including lipedema. You can achieve this by naturally burning fat. This ancestral mechanism of our body has been switched off with modern and infinite access to carbohydrates and can be activated with a simple dietary strategy.

We were all born with the instinct to eat a diet rich in nutrients and healthy fats. Still, too much conflicting information, commercial values, and access to nutritionally poor (but addictively tasty) food have led us to the most easily accessible energy: carbohydrates.

The ketogenic diet has been studied for decades. It is increasingly impressive for its therapeutic qualities, but it is still widely mistrusted by healthcare professionals who have not studied it thoroughly.

Indeed, you have heard this before: The key to everything is to eat fewer carbohydrates and more fats. But how do we balance this with the current but conflicting guidelines, which suggest up to 60% carbohydrates in the diet? Who is right?

Here, you will find the necessary strategies and 77 more ketogenic recipes to combine fat and protein consumption healthily. You will see how to lose weight and that getting healthy is much easier and tastier than you might think.

Based on decades of clinical studies and the extraordinary results he observed in patients he advised to stop eating carbohydrates, Dr. Alexandre Amato presents compelling arguments against the omnipresence of carbohydrates in today's diet.

The Ketogenic Therapy for Lipedema is easy to follow, simple to maintain, and clinically proven.

Easy to read, thought-provoking, and backed up by careful research, *Ketogenic Therapy for Lipedema* presents a dietary tactic that is light-hearted for laypeople and in-depth for health professionals;

through a new perspective, it is vitally essential for the most worrying health problems of our time.

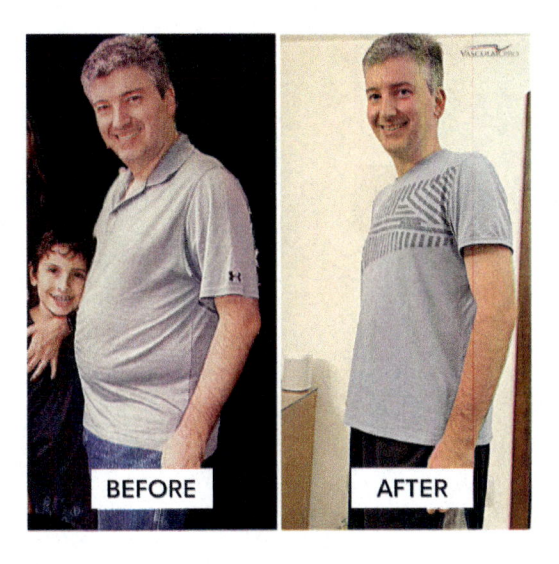

Alexandre Amato is a vascular surgeon with a doctorate in health sciences from USP (University of São Paulo) and a professor of medicine; he began applying the ketogenic diet to himself, obtaining excellent results at three points in his life. He started his nutritional studies, which eventually led to the book *Strategic Anti-Inflammatory Diet*, a first-line tactic in the symptomatic control of lipedema. He continued applying the method to his lipedema patients and was impressed with the results. Hence, he verified the consistency of the effects in patients with typical complaints from the vascular clinic and confirmed the importance of diet in clinical outcomes. The fear of dieting permeated today's society and made him delve deeper into the science behind this dietary change. Dr. Alexandre Amato is the creator of the best Brazilian health channel on YouTube (https://bio.amato.io/youtube) and a scientific researcher with international recognition (https://bio.amato.io/scholar), currently with a line of research focused on lipedema, a disease whose ketogenic diet has shown remarkable positive impact.

Index

Acknowledgments 12
Introduction 14
The ketogenic diet and its general principles 15
History of the ketogenic diet 19
Ketogenic alternatives and variations 23
    Supplements 24
    Atkins Diet 25
    Modified Atkins Diet 30
    Low-glycemic index diet 33
    Carnivore diet 37
    Low-carb diet 38
    Paleolithic diet 44
    Mediterranean Diet 47
    Intermittent fasting 48
    Commercial ketogenic diets 51
    Important considerations 54
Side effects of the ketogenic diet 58
Ketogenic diet and exercise 61
Uses of the ketogenic diet beyond epilepsy 62
    Lipedema 62
Effect of ketones 68
The ketogenic diet for weight loss 73
    Physiology of ketosis 75
Does the ketogenic diet work? 81
Other benefits in obesity 82

The yo-yo or accordion effect..83
Is the ketogenic diet safe?..85
Hypotheses on the mechanism of action of the ketogenic diet.......88
    The pH hypothesis 88
    Metabolic hypotheses 88
Healthy fats..89
    The Functions of Fats 89
    Different fats.. 89
How do you start the ketogenic diet in practice?...........................94
    Choice of food: 94
    How to prepare ketogenic meals quickly.............................. 100
    What is the best cooking oil?.. 101
    Is intermittent fasting necessary?.. 102
    How many meals should I eat a day? 102
    How long does it take to get into ketosis? 103
    What will I feel during the adaptation phase? 103
    How do I know if I'm in ketosis?.. 104
    How long should I follow the ketogenic diet?..................... 105
    How do you correctly read the nutritional table of foods? . 107
Conclusion: 118
Other books by the author..120
Ketogenic recipes...125
    Breakfast 125
    Lunch 147
    Dinner 163
    Desserts.. 186
Final message..207

Bibliography 209

Acknowledgments

Scientific research into diets without pharmaceutical intervention does not have the financial support of large companies. Because they have many variables and a lack of standardization, they are complex to carry out, compare, and maintain for a long time. Moreover, they do not offer anyone a direct financial return. The search for a patentable and saleable drug to solve a health problem can be much more seductive than the scientific study of a dietary strategy that has existed since homo sapiens appeared. Researchers are, therefore, generous souls who should be recognized. This book only has a scientific basis because of those who came before me and studied the subject. So, thank you to all the scientists who have dedicated themselves to studying the ketogenic diet and published their efforts and results, allowing others to delve deeper into the subject.

I would like to thank my wife, who had the patience to gently warn me that I was putting on more weight than was healthy and had the wisdom to wait for my acceptance of the problem, which was much slower than expected. He was with me two of the three times I went on the extended ketogenic diet, accepting, participating, and encouraging me. Even more, I am grateful for his companionship, love, and dedication, depriving himself of many moments by my side for the sake of this work and the revision of this book.

I would like to thank my mother, who not only encouraged me and provided me with the necessary education, as she is a cardiologist, but also proofread the content of this book with scientific rigor.

To my children, Guilherme and Sofia, who sacrificed the immediate gratification of their time with Dad so that I could finish this project, with the potential to increase our time together – should the increased longevity proposed by the ketogenic diet materialize.

I would like to thank my patients, who provided me with invaluable information and tips for practicing my diet daily.

I would like to thank everyone who helped make this book.

Introduction

Ketosis is a revolutionary and ancestral metabolic pathway capable of bringing numerous benefits to health, such as modulating inflammation, reducing oxidative stress, increasing histone acetylation, regulating mitophagy, inducing cellular redox status, and other mechanisms. The central nervous system cannot use fats directly as an energy source, so after 3 to 4 days without carbohydrate consumption, it is forced to find an alternative energy source. The ketones produced during ketosis have been called the brain's "super fuel," which is why ketogenic diets (which aim for ketosis) are of particular interest to neurology and have also been studied in oncology. Many cancers contain mitochondrial defects that make them dependent on glucose and certain hormones suppressed during ketosis. I must say in advance that the ketogenic diet will not be a definitive treatment or cure for any cancer, but it will probably be a powerful coadjuvant.

This book will tell you many things about the ketogenic diet. You can use this book as a resource for your health and the health of others. It is written in lay terms so that everyone can understand it without requiring complex science on the reader's part. Despite this, science was not left aside. The information contained herein is based on scientific literature, which we have appended to the bibliography that can be found at the end of this book.

The ketogenic diet and its general principles

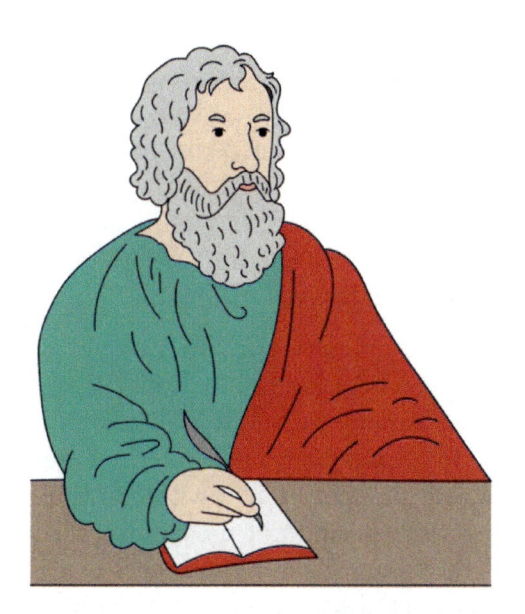

Hippocrates, 377 BC

"Let food be thy medicine, and let medicine be thy food."

Diet control is the oldest and most common way of treating diseases. The ketogenic diet has been known in medicine for a hundred years. It consists of eating high amounts of healthy fats, low carbohydrates, and adequate protein. Due to the large number of ketogenic variations, we can consider ketogenic diets as a category consisting of several different diets and strategies but with one common goal: the induction of a state of ketosis to a greater or lesser degree.

It is currently recognized and used to treat and control epileptic episodes in children[1,2], is beneficial in reducing amyloid plaques in Alzheimer's[3], reducing inflammation and fat in lipedema[4], controlling glycemia in type 2 diabetes[5], and as a coadjuvant hindering the proliferation of cancer cells[6–8], softening the impact of autism[9,10], improving motor dexterity in Parkinson's[11,12] resolving migraines[13,14], inducing lymphangiogenesis in lymphedema[15], improving mitochondrial function in multiple sclerosis[16], decreasing the action of IGF-1 on the skin and, consequently, acne[17], reducing insulin and IGF-1, improving polycystic ovary syndrome[17], etc. In other words, it is a dietary strategy used extensively in treating some diseases and is helpful in many other medical conditions. A beneficial tactic in so many illnesses would also be considered in situations of total health. At this point, it has positively impacted mood swings and improved quality of life[18].

Unfortunately, the main challenge of the ketogenic diet lies in its significant variability of strategies, the difficulty of carrying out extensive studies over long periods, complicated monitoring, limited adherence to the diet, and the lack of financial subsidies for comprehensive studies. Science is its own enemy by demanding an almost prohibitive strictness and not providing sufficient incentives to delve deeper into some issues in which there is no direct financial return. However, none of these factors that hinder science prevent personal use of this information. After all, the significant variability of the ketogenic diet offers several alternatives you can best identify. The necessary monitoring of ketosis for scientific research is often replaced by the quickly learned sensation of ketosis.

Unlike other diets, this one causes significant metabolic changes that affect every cell in the body, even before weight changes. On a ketogenic diet, paying attention to which foods you eat and which you should avoid is essential. You should eat foods that are high in fat but low in carbohydrates and moderate in protein. On a ketogenic diet, the body first uses its stored glucose for energy, but when it runs out of it, it turns to fat for energy. By breaking down the fat you eat and the fat you store, ketone bodies or ketones are energy molecules used as fuel for your activities. When you use ketones as your primary fuel instead of glucose, you are in a state of ketosis. On the other hand, foods rich in carbohydrates are easily transformed into glucose. Around 90 to 100% of ingested carbohydrates are converted quickly and effortlessly into glucose and enter the bloodstream.

So, if you want to enter a state of ketosis, gradually reduce the amount of carbohydrates you eat and increase the amount of fats. Remember that the most common foods contain carbohydrates and should be avoided. These include pasta, bread, cereals, milkshakes, potatoes, rice and most sweets.

To accurately track the amount of carbohydrates in each meal, you should consistently record your food intake, be responsible for selecting and buying your food, and meticulously plan or monitor every bite you take. By doing so, you can avoid situations where you have no suitable food alternatives, ensuring precise management of your carbohydrate consumption.

Remember that before starting any diet, you should always consult your doctor, especially if you are unsure about your health problems. This is particularly important if you have diabetes, thyroid dysfunction, autoimmune diseases, intestinal problems, vitamin and mineral deficiencies, or if you are pregnant or breastfeeding.

Therefore, in the ketogenic diet, carbohydrates should be avoided. They can be found in grains composed predominantly of carbohydrates (wheat, rice, corn, oats, rye, barley, and others) and their derived products, such as pasta, bread, pies, and cake. Also, avoid most fruits that naturally contain sugar (fructose). Also, prevent root vegetables such as carrots, turnips, potatoes, beans, and legumes. They have a lot of starch. Do not consume sugar. Avoid milk and skimmed or semi-skimmed products, as these contain more carbohydrates than fats. Sugarcane is grass, and its sweet taste is due to the high concentration of sugar, so no more sugarcane juice or brown sugar candy.

A ketogenic diet, based on current evidence, is safe for the general population and can be considered the first choice in cases of obesity and diabetes[18]. To successfully enter ketosis, it's advised to consume no more than 20 grams of carbohydrates daily for four weeks. You can then increase your intake by 5 grams per week until you reach the individual maximum (approximately 40 grams) to maintain ketosis[19]. The ketosis state can be identified by metallic or bad breath (ketosis breath); it can increase the urge to urinate, consequently increase thirst, decrease hunger, and cause headaches, nausea, and weakness. During ketosis, some people may also experience a state of euphoria and improved mental acuity. If you have a ketone meter and want to use it, a measurement between 0.5 and 3 mmol/L suggests that you have reached a state of ketosis. The most accurate way to identify ketosis is a blood test, but in the practice of dieting, the test is not necessary.

As of the date this was written, the website clinicaltrials.gov lists 302 active studies focused on the ketogenic diet. Medicine is a changing science, and we must understand that new evidence can alter previous theories.

History of the ketogenic diet.

The ketogenic diet was developed in the early 1920s for epileptic children and fell out of favor in the 1970s and 1980s with the introduction of drug treatments for epilepsy. However, we can trace its history even in the Bible, in the healing of the demon-possessed boy[i]. The difficulty of maintaining a strict diet, the lack of a broad understanding of how diet works in epilepsy, and the commercial appeal of drugs have led the market to drugs that are easier to access. The medications had a well-explained theory of pathophysiology, at least from a theoretical point of view, and this was comfortable for the prescriber. Despite this, in 1996, the diet's reputation resurfaced with the American Epilepsy Association.

Today, even with new drugs, it is known that ketosis induced by the ketogenic diet can be more effective than many drugs still in use[20]. The diet had an impact on difficult-to-control epileptic seizures, paving the way for the study of ketosis in other medical conditions. New insights into the mechanism of action have led to a better understanding of brain metabolism and, thus, the control of epilepsy.

In the 1920s, treatment with bromides and phenobarbital was incapacitating, with a high sedative effect. Hugh Conklin believed that toxic substances caused epilepsy in the brain from the intestines. He postulated that by letting the intestine rest, the intoxication would be reduced, and he ended up introducing food fasting for 25 days as a treatment. At that time, he deprived the children of all food, allowing only water. In 1922, he showed a high remission rate, with many children free of epileptic episodes for long periods. Its success was spread even before official scientific publication. This hope led to much research into the workings and interrelationships of fat, protein, and carbohydrate metabolism. At the time, the ketone bodies caused by fasting were identified as the immediate result of the

---

[i] New Testament, Matthew, 17:14-21, "However, this kind does not go out except by prayer and fasting".

oxidation of fatty acids in the absence of glucose, and it was postulated that they had anticonvulsant effects.

Although prolonged fasting was challenging for severe epileptics, it was still considered much better than frequent episodes of events. In 1921, Wilder published the first article on the high-fat, low-carbohydrate diet at the Mayo Clinic. A diet that provided protein for growth, minimal carbohydrates, and the rest in fats[2]. This diet was very close to the ketogenic diet we have today. With reports and subsequent work until 1938, when the drug phenytoin appeared, and from then on, academic attention was diverted to the action of the new anticonvulsant chemicals. In the years that followed, with the decline in attention to diet and the focus on medication, diet was gradually forgotten, and the ability to apply it in practice was lost. Nutritionists were less in demand to apply the diet. After all, it was easier to prescribe a drug than to institute a restrictive and challenging diet at the time, which required rigor and commitment from the patient and their family. Over time, professionals lost the ability to prescribe the diet, and it was often applied incorrectly and ineffectively, with frustrating results. The knowledge and skills acquired at the start of the revolution were lost. With this inability, an entire generation saw and propagated the diet as difficult to tolerate and incapable of bringing good results. However, at the end of the 1980s, it was realized that when properly applied, in severe cases, the diet's success rate was as good as the original description. At the famous *Johns Hopkins* Hospital in the 1990s, the diet was applied to around ten children yearly. With the appearance in the media of the treatment of some illustrious people, there has been greater awareness of the problem. The emergence of foundations to publicize the technique and even films, such as "First Do No Harm" with Meryl Streep in 1997, once again stimulated studies, and a large multicenter study was presented in 1996 with 150 patients.[21]

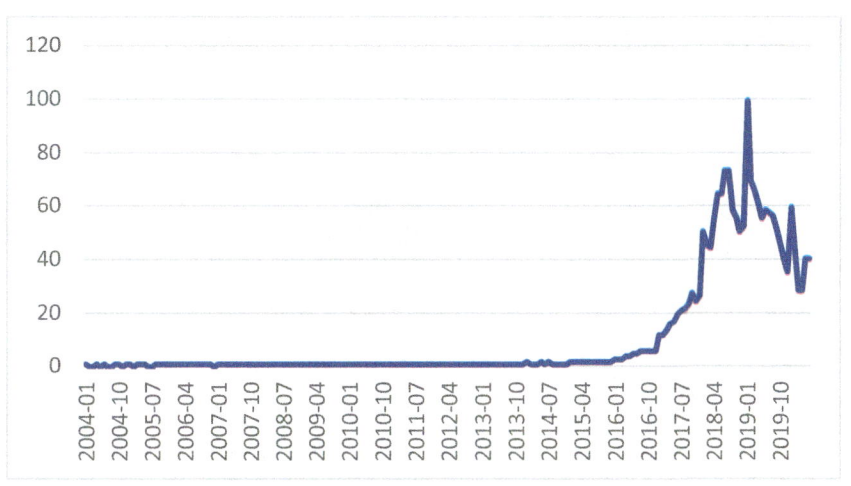

Figure 1 - Google Trends interest in ketogenic diet

It is really impressive that something with such a positive impact discovered decades ago has remained in scientific limbo for so long. I imagine that the lack of funding from big pharmaceutical companies, for obvious reasons, covered up this therapeutic tool during this period. But we cannot ignore the influence of the food market, which is eager to sell carbohydrates that promote the neurochemical effect of food addiction[22].

From the point of view of globalization, the ketogenic diet took a long time to reach the world, probably due to cultural, financial, and religious reasons.

Over the years, advances in understanding metabolism have led to minor but impactful changes and evolutions in the original concept of diets, enhancing their effectiveness and simplicity. This evolution has expanded their applicability. Recent studies indicate that initiating diets with an average calorie count, without an initial fasting period, is effective. Consequently, hospitalization, which was once necessary to start the diet, especially for children, is no longer required. Despite these advancements in physiological knowledge, the exact mechanism by which the ketogenic diet functions as an anticonvulsant remains not fully understood.

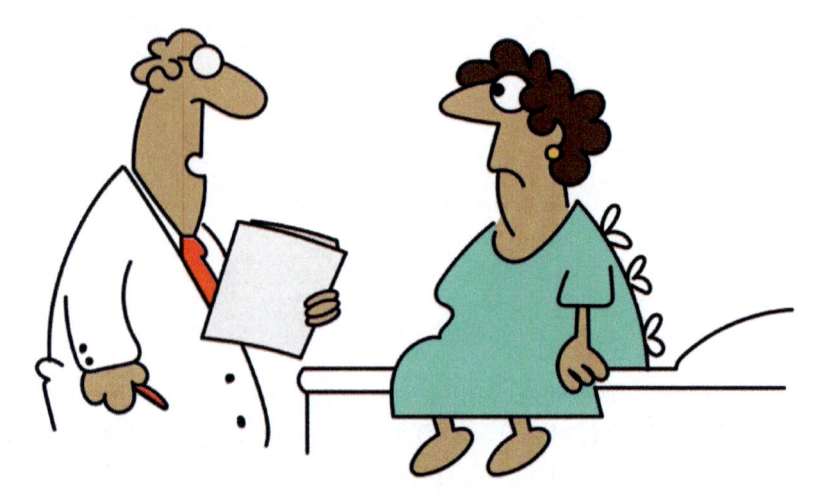

Ketogenic Therapy for Lipedema, by Alexandre Amato

"The carbohydrate diet that I prescribed for you 20 years ago led to diabetes, high blood pressure and atherosclerosis. My bad..."

Ketogenic alternatives and variations

Considering that the primary definition of ketogenic diets is the proportion of proteins, fats, and carbohydrates, many diets can fit into the definition of ketogenic despite having other names. By getting to know the ketogenic alternatives, you will discover the pattern behind them and understand their essence. You will realize that the basic principle is always the same, but the way of streamlining the process is different. The hypothalamus produces a hormone called oxytocin, which is responsible, among other things, for creating empathy between people. Through this creation of empathy, it is possible to make people feel the need to help others. However, for this hormone to be produced by the brain, attention must first be created. Otherwise, the audience will not be interested in the narrative, and consequently, their brains will not produce the substance that provokes empathy. It is crucial to have a positive first approach that captures the audience's attention so that the brain can produce a hormone called cortisol before oxytocin. This increases our attention and focus so that we can create empathy with the unfolding of the story. The human brain identifies with stories about complex challenges and consecutive triumphs.

Some people are persuaded by the narrative of a carnivorous or paleolithic diet, which I must agree with; they are contagious logic. Other people are satisfied with lists of foods they can and cannot eat without further context. Some are more systematic and need a convincing and in-depth technical explanation based on much prestigious science. Others need multi-professional support with someone telling them what they can and cannot do, constantly getting them back on track. The good news is that the ketogenic diet has all this in its alternatives and variations. You just need to find the mode you like best.

Supplements

Medium-chain triglycerides (MCTs)[ii], derived from certain foods, are nothing more than processed fats with a smaller molecular size, providing faster metabolization and, therefore, comparable to the speed at which carbohydrates are broken down. Long-chain triglycerides, commonly consumed in the traditional diet, are slowly absorbed. Adding MCTs to your diet does not make it a ketogenic diet, but it is possible to add MCTs oils to increase ketone bodies and enhance the benefits of ketosis. Studies have shown that regular use of MCTs can be beneficial in preventing and controlling obesity, atherosclerosis, and diabetes[22,23].

[ii] Medium-chain triglycerides (MCTs) are molecules formed by three saturated fatty acids with a length of 6 to 12 carbon atoms esterified with glycerol. Specifically, they are caprylic (C8:0), caproic (C6:0), capric (C10:0) and lauric (C12:0) acids. Foods rich in TCMs include coconut oil (58%), palm oil (54%), dried coconut (37%) and raw coconut meat (19%).

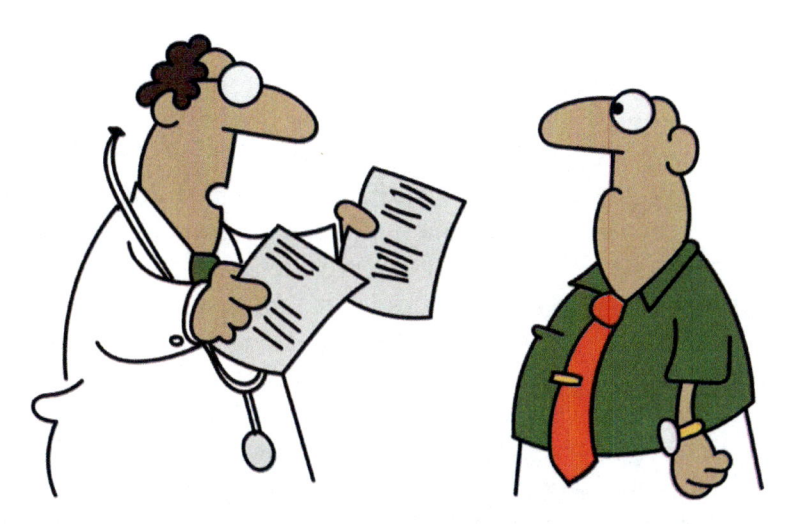

"On this diet you can eat as much meat as you want, but one slice of bread will kill you. In this other one you can eat as much bread as you want, but a steak will kill you."

Atkins Diet

Dr. Robert Atkins described the diet that bears his name in 1972 in his book "Dr. Atkins' Diet Revolution," restricting the amount of carbohydrates to 10 to 20 g per day. The Atkins diet induces ketosis without limiting protein, fluids, or calories and without requiring fasting or hospitalization. In his time, Atkins created an obesity treatment center in New York. The diet drastically reduces the intake of carbohydrates, with 98% of the daily calories ingested consisting of proteins and animal fats. According to Atkins, when you start the diet, the body's metabolism changes so that it starts using body fat for energy instead of carbohydrates. In this process, also known as ketosis, the body is induced not to feel hungry, as there is no limit to calorie consumption. Atkins recommends eating until you feel sufficiently satisfied without feeling "stuffed." This helps control binge eating and induces weight loss. Taking multivitamins is essential for a successful diet. The Atkins diet was cited in 89,000 articles in a Google Scholar[iii] search. According to the first reports, when he died in 2003 at 72, Atkins weighed 116kg and was 1.8m tall[iv]. Obviously, the rumor spread that he died from his own diet[v], giving the ketogenic diet a bad name. I remember it clearly because his death occurred the year I started my residency in general surgery, and the commentary in medical circles was always negative about the diet. However, his medical history later came to light: he developed cardiomyopathy in 2000 as a result of a viral illness, which led to a heart attack two years later. The direct cause of death was a fall when he slipped on ice on his way to work on foot, I repeat, at the age of 72. The hospital admission records state that he weighed 88 kg at the time. His weight at the time of death of 116 kg was probably due to anasarca[vi] contracted during a two-week stay in the intensive care unit. His death certificate states that the cause of death was "blunt impact injury to the head with epidural hematoma." The actual cause of Dr. Atkins' death, according to medical reports, was a head injury he suffered, not the diet program he created. Apparently, opponents of the vegan group spread falsehoods about his death, but the mainstream media accelerated this process of fake news, a term that didn't exist at the time. In March 2007, Newsweek magazine published a correction: "An earlier version of this story contained an inaccurate succession of events surrounding the death of Dr. Robert Atkins. Newsweek regrets the error."

[iii] https://scholar.google.com is a freely accessible virtual search engine that organizes and lists full text or metadata of academic literature in a wide variety of publication formats. Google Scholar has been criticized for not vetting publications and including predatory journals in its index.
[iv] https://bio.amato.io/atkins1
[v] https://bio.amato.io/atkins2
[vi] Anasarca is a state of generalized edema present in various diseases, the most frequent being heart failure, cirrhosis and nephrotic syndrome.

Atkins Diet

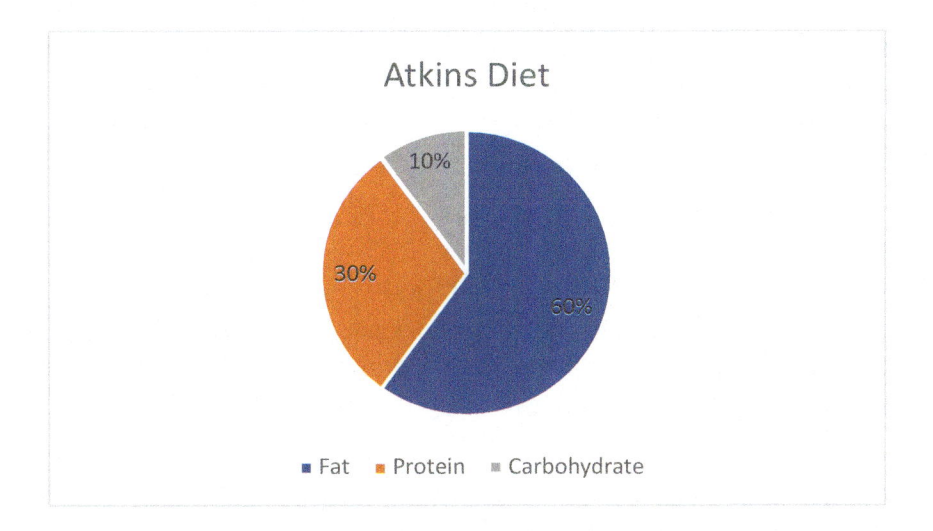

- Fat: 60%
- Protein: 30%
- Carbohydrate: 10%

The Atkins diet consists of 4 steps:

Ketosis induction

For 15 days, the diet should not exceed a daily intake of 20g of carbohydrates. The diet is restricted to animal proteins, eggs, fish, and seafood. This period is recommended to induce the metabolism into ketosis and prepare it for the more extended diet phase. Remember that in some cases, it is also recommended to remain at this stage until the weight to be reduced is less than 16 kg. Below this weight to be lost, moving on to the next stage is recommended. Otherwise, the ideal is 15 days of induction, two days of eating regular carbohydrates (without overdoing it), and then another 15 days of induction. And so on until less than 16 kg have been lost.

Continued weight loss

This stage is the most extended period that will lead to continued weight loss. Atkins introduces yellow cheeses, sour cream, and some types of nuts in moderation. It also suggests eating more vegetables. Advising to avoid caffeine and aspartame[vii] (coffee, Coca-Cola zero sugar).

[vii] Aspartame is a food additive used as a substitute for ordinary sugar and was created in 1965. It has greater sweetening power (around 200 times sweeter than

Pre-maintenance

You must move to this stage when the desired weight is reached. The carbohydrate limit here increases to 100g, which allows you to eat bread and legumes. This period aims to prepare the person for maintenance.

Maintenance

In the final period, the person will find a balance in how much carbohydrate they can eat. This value varies from 200g to 500g. Atkins recommends monitoring your weight monthly and suggests that you can eat more carbohydrates by exercising.

Criticism

Contrary to modern nutrition and the consensual and established food pyramid (Figure 5), Atkins was harshly criticized for decades by medical and food institutions.

The diet was also widely criticized in medical circles for recommending an intake of saturated fats[viii] of animal origin and radically reducing the intake of carbohydrates, especially those with a high glycemic index. Medical associations recommended against the diet. Meanwhile, Atkins' business continued to thrive, delivering results. At the end of the 1980s, the Atkins Center was opened in New York, where he brought together dozens of doctors, nutritionists, and scientists who supported him and led patients through implementing the diet.

In 2003, some doctors decided for the first time to carry out a controlled study on the diet, comparing it to conventional diets recommended by medical associations (high in carbohydrates and

---

sucrose) and is less dense. It is usually sold added to other products and is the sweetener most commonly used in drinks.

[viii]Saturated fat is one of the types of fat present in foods. It differs from unsaturated fat in that there is no double bond between two neighboring carbon atoms in a fatty acid chain. That is, the chain is completely "saturated" with hydrogen atoms. During the 20th century, with the growing obesity epidemic, studies were carried out which apparently linked the consumption of saturated fat to an increase in cholesterol levels.

low in fat and calories) [24]. Surprisingly, the diet performed better not only in reducing weight but also in reducing body fat (percentage) and improving lipid and glycemic profiles in basically all the groups studied—nevertheless, adherence to the diet without professional monitoring results in nutritional deficiencies. New studies have been carried out on low-carbohydrate diets, and their results are always more favorable regarding weight loss, fat loss, and improved blood profiles[25].

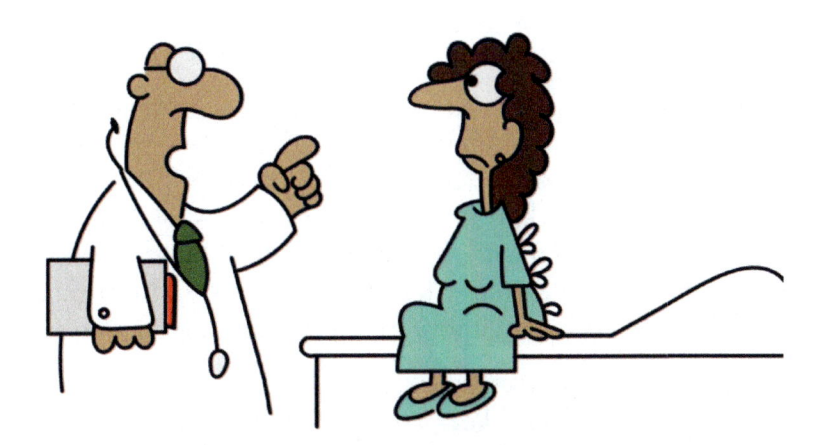

"You did the Atkins diet and lost 40 kilos, lowered your cholesterol, cured your high blood pressure, and now you run 8 km a day. But I'm warning you, the ketogenic diet is bad for your health."

Modified Atkins Diet

The principles of the modified Atkins diet are more accessible to follow and implement. There is no formal list for food composition except for carbohydrates. No specification of carbohydrates can or cannot be eaten, but those with a low glycemic index (berries and whole grains) allow more carbohydrates to be eaten. Modified Atkins and the low-glycemic index diet differ in the amount and type of carbohydrates consumed. Sugars, flour, and cereals are not part of the modified Atkins diet. Protein sources include red meat (beef or pork), white meat (chicken or fish), and eggs. Fats are offered in fresh cream, mayonnaise, cream, coconut milk, bacon, and vegetable oils. The modified Atkins diet is discussed in 29,000 articles in the academic search system Google Scholar.

Start

It starts with laboratory tests (lipid profile, fasting glucose, liver enzymes, vitamins, and minerals) and a 2-day food record. High-fat foods are added. Carbohydrates: 10g/day for children, 15g/day for adolescents, and 20g/day for adults (net carbs = total carbs - fiber). Add multivitamins and calcium supplements with vitamin D daily. If available and possible, add a KetoCal® 4:1 shake (400 calories) in the first month. Liquids without carbohydrates are encouraged.

Monitoring and maintenance (1st month)

Weight should be checked weekly. Ketone bodies should be measured twice a week for at least the first month. You should also measure the amount of carbohydrates you eat using tables, apps, and guides. Do not change anticonvulsant medication. Avoid artificial carbohydrate-free products.

Maintenance (after the 1st month)

You can increase the amount of carbohydrates (5 to 10g/day), change anticonvulsants, and use low-carb products. Reevaluate laboratory tests, including a lipid profile, after three months. Food record after three months.

Closing

Increase the carbohydrate limit by 10g per day for up to 60g/day, then replace it with regular food once a week.

Table 1 - Differences between the ketogenic diet and the modified Atkins diet

	Classic ketogenic diet (Figure 2)	Modified Atkins diet (Figure 4)
Calories (% recommended daily allowance)	Restricted (75%) or maintained	Not restricted
Liquids	Daily recommendation	Not restricted
Fat	85-90%	~60%
Protein	15%	~30%
Carbohydrates	5%	~10%
Fasting period	Occasional	Not used
Hospital assessment	Frequent	No
Heavy and measured food	Yes	No
Sharing food with family	No	Yes
Option of eating in restaurants	No	Yes
Industrialized low-carb foods	Not used	Allowed sporadically
Nutritionist involvement	Yes	Usually yes
Scientific studies	Yes	Yes

Classic 4:1 Ketogenic Diet

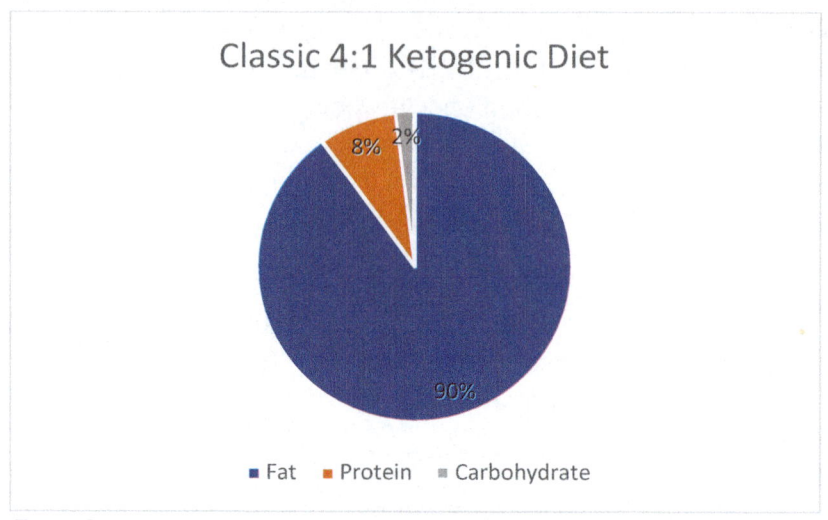

- Fat 90%
- Protein 8%
- Carbohydrate 2%

Figure 2 - *Proportion of macronutrients in the classic ketogenic diet (4:1)*

Classic 3:1 Ketogenic Diet

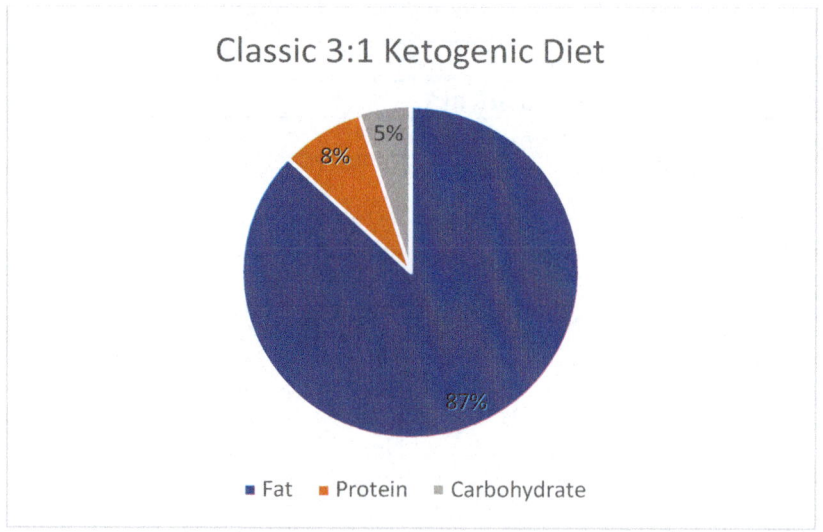

- Fat 87%
- Protein 8%
- Carbohydrate 5%

Figure 3 - Proportion of macronutrients in the classic ketogenic diet[13]

Modified Atkins Diet

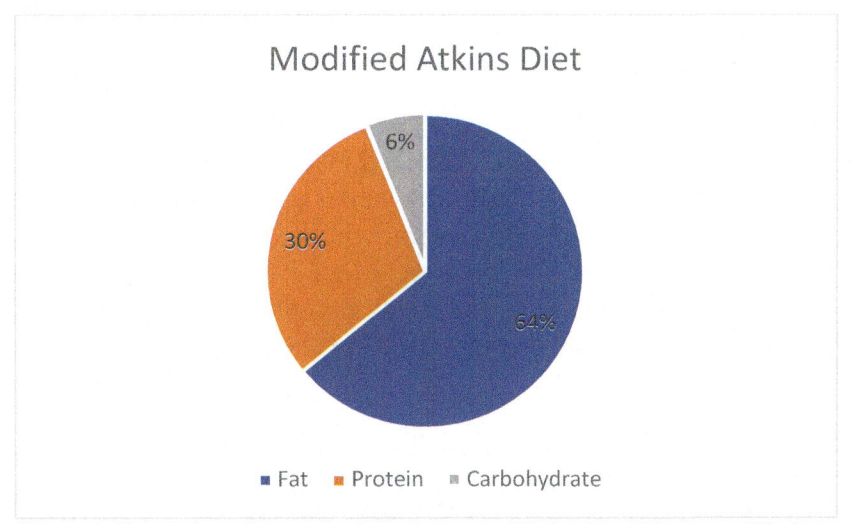

[Pie chart: Fat 64%, Protein 30%, Carbohydrate 6%]

Figure 4 - Proportion of macronutrients in the modified Atkins Diet or modified ketogenic diet[13]

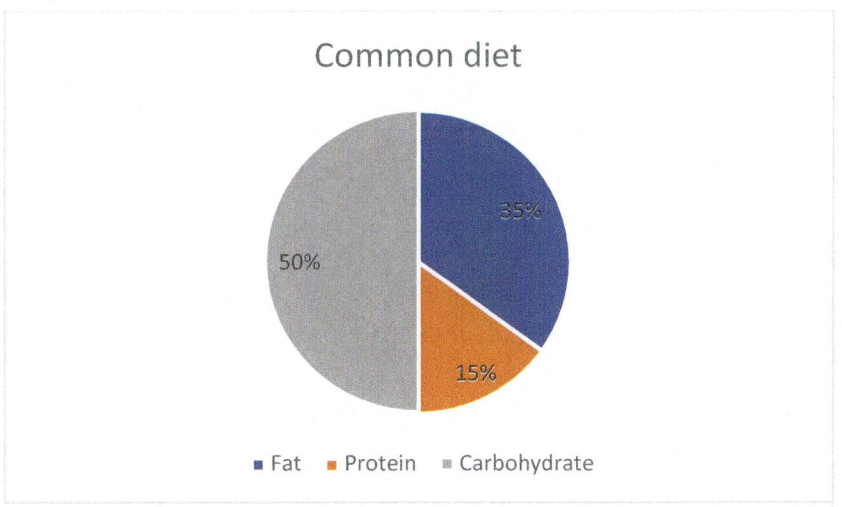

Common diet

[Pie chart: Fat 35%, Protein 15%, Carbohydrate 50%]

Figure 5 - Proportion of macronutrients in the typical diet

Low-glycemic index diet

The low-glycemic index diet discourages fruits, pasta, and starches. It has fewer carbohydrates than the Atkins diet (Figure 6). The aim of low-glycemic index diets is not to form ketone bodies but to keep the glycemic index low. However, it also affects other metabolites[25], suggesting improvements in several diseases, such as obesity, diabetes, cardiovascular disease, and some types of cancer.

The glycemic index represents the speed at which the carbohydrate is digested and finally transformed into sugar in the blood. When you consume foods with a high glycemic index, i.e., those that are digested more quickly, your blood sugar levels rise rapidly, and you need to release more insulin to normalize your blood sugar levels. This situation can overload the pancreas and lead to insulin resistance and even diabetes.

When sugar levels rise excessively, there is a greater tendency for the body to store fat, favoring weight gain.

Foods with slow-digesting carbohydrates release sugar in smaller quantities, or at a slower rate, into the bloodstream and are, therefore, low on the glycemic index. These foods are fiber-rich, making us feel fuller and help us lose weight. Your food intake will decrease since you need to eat less to feel satisfied.

The glycemic index diet considers the type of food eaten, prioritizing the consumption of foods with a low glycemic index.

A meta-analysis of 54 studies showed that low-glycemic index diets have laboratory and body mass index (BMI)[ix] benefits in patients with insulin resistance and diabetes.[25]. There is an improvement in low-density lipoprotein (LDL[x]) and triglycerides and an increase in

---

[ix] The body mass index (BMI) is an international measure used to calculate whether a person is at their ideal weight. BMI is determined by dividing an individual's mass by the square of their height, where mass is in kilograms and height is in meters.

[x] Low-density lipoprotein (LDL) is part of the lipoprotein family. It is popularly called bad cholesterol because at high levels it is related to atherosclerosis and is therefore also indirectly related to heart attacks and strokes. In general, LDL transports cholesterol and triglycerides from the liver and small intestine to the cells and tissues that need these substances.

high-density lipoprotein (HDL[xi]). Inflammatory markers such as C-reactive protein and interleukin-6 also decrease.

The low-glycemic index diet is cited in 6 thousand articles on Google Scholar.

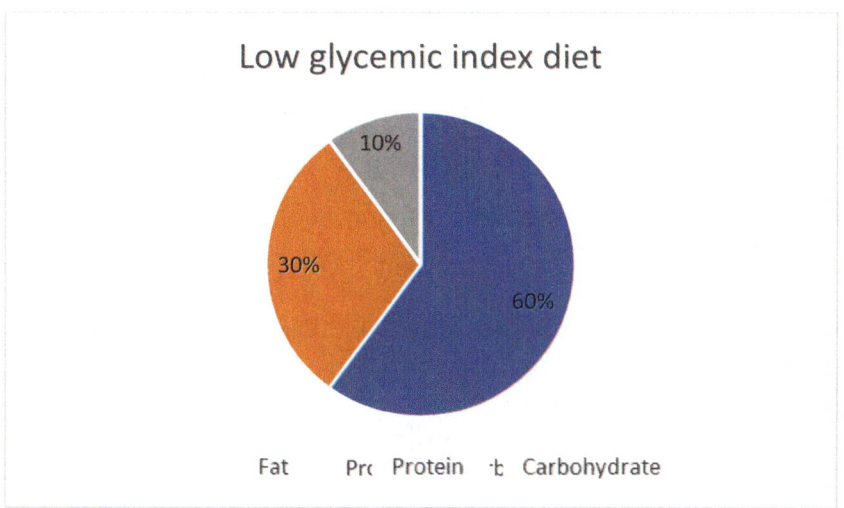

Figure 6 - Low-glycemic index diet[13]

Low-glycemic index foods that can be consumed:
In general, foods that are high in fiber have lower glycemic ratings. The fibrous coatings around grains and seeds mean the body breaks them down more slowly. Therefore, they tend to be lower on the glycemic scale than foods without this coating. But cooking time also influences the glycemic index: the longer a food is cooked, the more it rises in the glycemic index. When food is cooked, the starch or carbohydrates begin to break down. Also, as a general rule, the more

---

[xi] High-density lipoprotein (HDL) is part of the lipoprotein family. It is called "good cholesterol" because it is believed to be able to remove atheromas from the arteries. HDL transports cholesterol from the tissues of the human body to the liver – this is called reverse cholesterol transport. This decreases blood and cellular cholesterol levels, reducing the risk of diseases caused by hypercholesterolemia, such as coronary artery disease, corneal opacities and planar xanthomas. HDL "receives" part of the cholesterol from LDL while "giving" apoproteins to it, thus making it easier for LDL to return to the liver and preventing it from remaining in the bloodstream.

processed a food is, the higher it is on the glycemic scale. For example, fruit juice has a higher glycemic index rating than fresh fruit. For example, highly acidic foods, such as pickles, tend to be lower on the glycemic index than non-acidic foods. In addition, the riper a fruit or vegetable, the higher its glycemic index tends to be. Although there are exceptions to every rule, these are some general guidelines to follow when assessing the potential impact of a specific food on blood sugar.

These are foods with a low glycemic index:

- **Fruits:** cherry, grapefruit, dried apricot, pear, apple, orange, red plum, strawberry, peach, grape, avocado, carambola, fig, guava, and tangerine.
- **Vegetables:** zucchini, chard, watercress, celery, lettuce, garlic, asparagus, eggplant, broccoli, alfalfa sprout, bamboo shoot, onion, spring onion, carrot, chicory, coriander, mushroom, cabbage, cauliflower, spinach, gilo, maroon cucumber, mustard, turnip, heart of palm, cucumber, bell pepper, okra, radish, cabbage, arugula, parsley, arrowleaf elephant's ear, tomato and green beans.
- **Beans:** kidney beans, lentils, peas, soybeans and chickpeas.
- **Meats:** lean, fat-free cuts, fish, and skinless chicken.
- Skimmed milk and dairy products.
- **Oilseeds:** walnuts, peanuts and chestnuts.
- Natural sweeteners such as fructose and stevia.

High glycemic index foods that cannot be consumed:

- Foods made with refined flours: pasta, French bread, cakes, and cookies.
- Refined sugar, brown sugar, honey, molasses, soft drinks and fruit juices.
- White rice, potatoes, and corn.
- Fruits: pineapple, banana, papaya, mango, watermelon, melon, raisins, persimmon, sweet fruit and kiwi.
- Artificial sweeteners: saccharin, cyclamate, and aspartame.

Carnivore diet

What would you say to a diet based solely on meat, offal, eggs, fish, and cured cheeses (Figure 7)? The carnivore diet is surprisingly the opposite of the vegan lifestyle: no vegetables, plant-based foods, or supplements. But there is another big difference: carbohydrates exist in much smaller quantities in the animal world, so it is a variation of the ketogenic diet. For example, one egg (100g) has 155 calories, 13g of protein, 11g of lipids and 1.1g of carbohydrates.

It is a version of a diet with a high protein and saturated fat content and no carbohydrates with a simple fundamental rule that directs food selection. However, there is no set protocol for the amount of proteins and fats to eat. While some variations of the carnivore diet allow whole dairy products, the most extreme followers omit dairy products altogether.

So, the carnivore diet is a more extreme version of the ketogenic diet and, as the name suggests, means eating only animal-based foods. The carnivorous ketogenic diet follows the carnivorous diet but can include non-animal but healthy fats and some fiber-rich fruits, vegetables, and dairy products.

The carnivore diet has almost 5 thousand articles on Google Scholar.

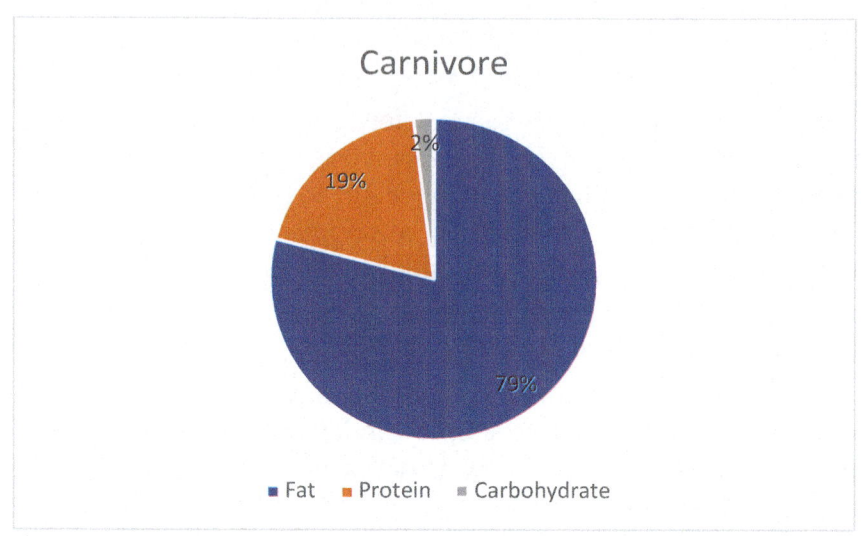

Figure 7 - Macronutrient distribution in the carnivore diet

Low-carb diet

The low-carb diet has been around for a long time and is still going strong. It requires you to reduce your intake of high-carb foods, such as bread, pasta, or tapioca, to increase your consumption of proteins, such as eggs, beef, chicken, and fish, as well as good quality fats from avocados, olive oil, and nuts, among other things (figure 6).

This diet is an option for losing weight due to the addition of more low-carb, high-fiber vegetables, such as chayote, spinach, or zucchini, and an increase in the amount of protein-rich foods, such as fish, eggs, or lean meats, and good fats that help reduce appetite.

Additionally, in the low-carb diet, regular intake of fruit, vegetables, and nuts, which are rich in antioxidants, vitamins, and minerals, helps to lower cholesterol, triglyceride, and blood sugar levels, preventing diseases such as stroke, diabetes, and obesity.

Processed foods rich in bad fats, such as bacon, French fries, ice cream, cookies, and alcoholic beverages, should be avoided, as these types of foods cause weight gain and contribute to the emergence of diseases such as cancer, hepatic steatosis, and obesity.

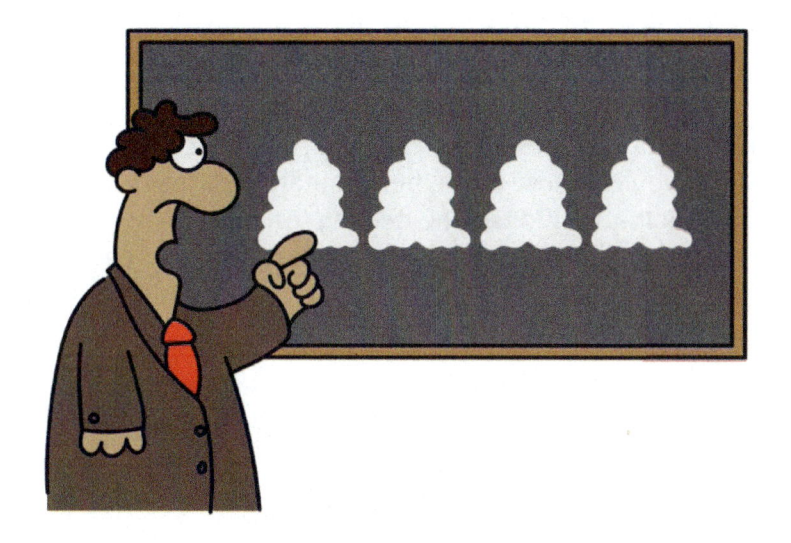

"These are the 4 white powders that are destroying our society: sugar, salt, wheat flour and cocaine."

To follow the low-carb diet, you should especially remove simple carbohydrates from your diet, such as sugar, white wheat flour, soft drinks, and sweets. Depending on the amount of carbohydrates in the diet, it may also be necessary to restrict the intake of some complex carbohydrates, such as bread, oats, rice, or pasta.

A "normal" diet generally consumes an average of 250 g of carbohydrates per day. On the low-carb diet, the objective is to ingest from 130 g to 200 g of carbohydrates per day, which is equivalent to approximately one medium banana + 200 g of full-fat natural yogurt + 2 tablespoons of oats + 2 tablespoons of honey, in the morning and afternoon snack, for example.

Since your body is accustomed to consuming a large amount of carbohydrates, it's advisable to gradually transition to a low-carb diet. This gradual change allows your body to adjust, reducing the likelihood of experiencing symptoms such as headaches, dizziness, or mood swings.

It is crucial to have three main meals and two snacks during the low-carb diet. So you eat more often, but in small portions throughout the day, which helps to reduce the feeling of hunger. Breakfast and snacks should include eggs, cheese, nuts, avocado, and coconut. Lunch and dinner should be rich in salad, protein, and olive oil and may contain just a few carbohydrates.

A low-carb diet may not work when you consider carbohydrate addiction, and, unlike a ketogenic diet, it does not lead the body into physiological ketosis.

The low-carb diet has almost 5 thousand articles on Google Scholar.

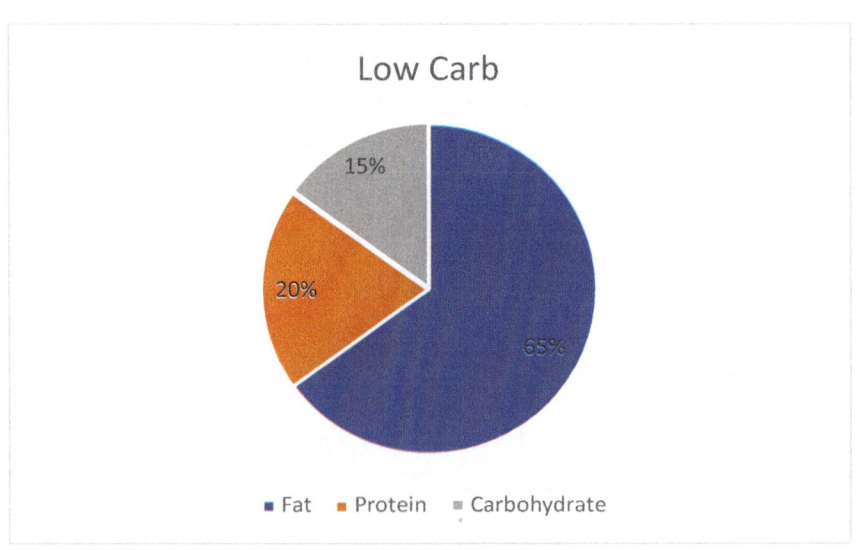

Figure 8 - Macronutrient distribution in the low-carb diet

Foods prohibited on the low-carb diet

It is essential to avoid high-carb foods on the low-carb diet, as they can negatively affect the diet. The types of food that should be avoided include:

- **Sugar:** refined sugar, soft drinks, processed fruit juices, sweeteners and sweets.
- **Cereals:** white rice, white pasta, farofa and couscous.
- **Dried fruits:** raisins, apricots and plums.
- **Flours:** tapioca, white wheat flour, and foods prepared with it, such as white bread, pancakes, cakes, and biscuits.

In addition to high-carb foods, it is also necessary to exclude industrialized foods such as pizza and cookies, those rich in bad fats such as margarine, ice cream, sausages, chips and bacon, and alcoholic drinks.

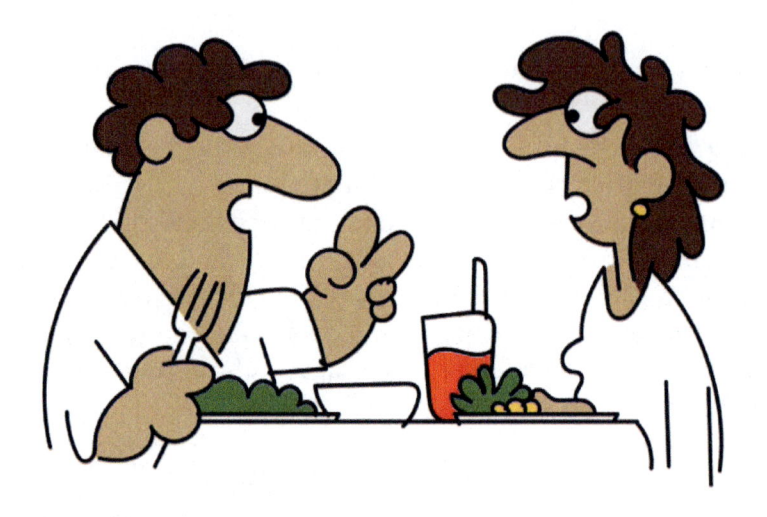

-I'm eating twice as many vegetables as before
-Two times zero is still zero

Foods allowed on the low-carb diet

The foods allowed on the low-carb diet are:

- **Fresh, whole fruits**, with peel and in small quantities, such as apple, lemon, kiwi, cashew, plum, guava, and papaya.
- **Vegetables in small quantities**, such as lettuce, arugula, tomatoes, chayote, and cauliflower.
- **Lean proteins**, especially skinless chicken or turkey.
- **Fish**, preferably fattier fish such as salmon, tuna, trout, and sardines.
- **Milk and dairy**, such as cheese and yogurt.
- **Good fats**, like olive oil, coconut oil, and butter.
- **Nuts**, such as walnuts, almonds, Brazil nuts, and peanuts.

- **Seeds in general**, such as chia, flaxseed, sunflower seeds, pumpkin seeds, and sesame.
- **Drinks**, such as unsweetened coffee and tea.

Milk can be replaced with coconut or almond milk, which has a much lower carbohydrate content. It is essential to add 2 to 3 liters of water per day.

Some foods with moderate amounts of carbohydrates, such as beans, lentils, brown rice, potatoes, cassava, sweet potatoes, yams, and pumpkin, can be included in the low-carb diet in some cases.

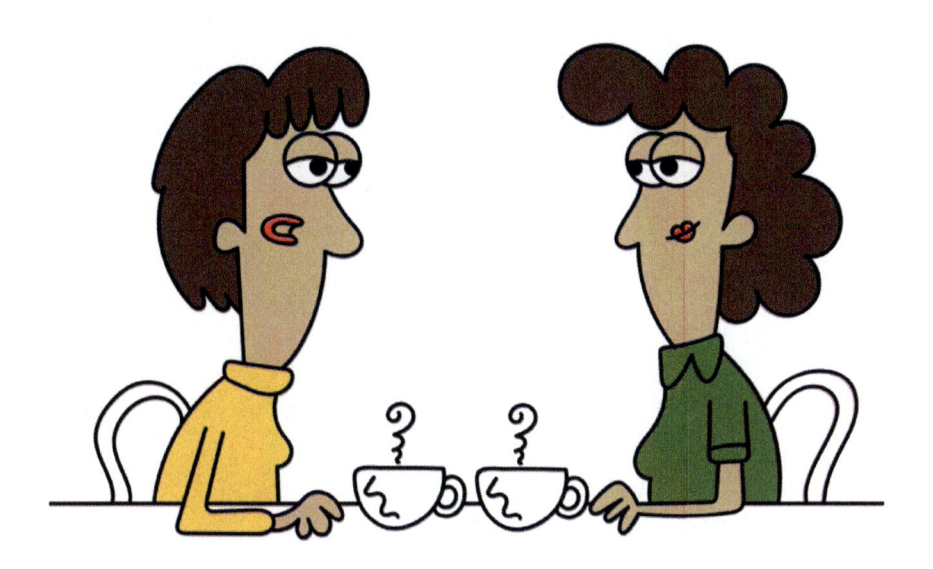

"It just wasn't working. He was a low-carb liberal and I'm a restricted ketogenic."

Paleolithic diet

The paleo or paleolithic diet is a diet consisting of food based on wild plants, meat, fish, and eggs, which were commonly consumed by Homo sapiens during the Paleolithic period[xii]. The period during which agriculture began to develop. It became popular in the mid-1970s thanks to gastroenterologist Walter L. Voegtlin. It is based on the premise that humans are genetically adapted to the diet of their Paleolithic ancestors and that there has been little genetic adaptation since the beginning of agriculture. Therefore, according to the theory, the ideal diet for human health and well-being should resemble that of their Paleolithic ancestors (Figure 9).

[xii] The Paleolithic or Chipped Stone Age is the first periodic phase of history, beginning around 2.5 million years ago and ending in 10,000 B.C. This period was marked by the development of oral and written communication, the creation of the first stone tools, and the use of fire by humans. Paleolithic (2.5 million - 10,000 BC)

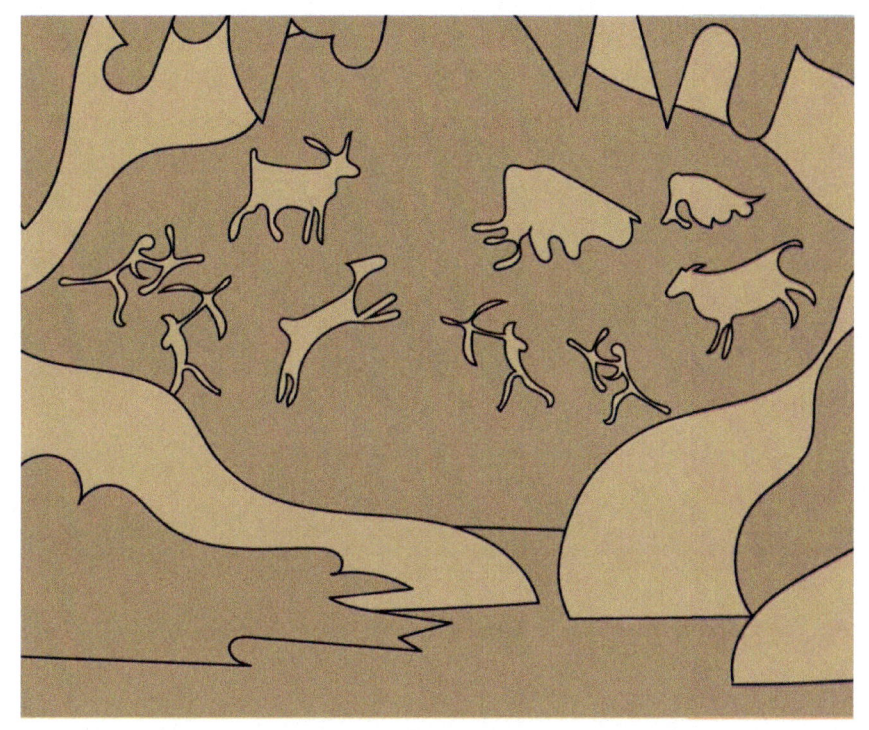

"We have never found a cave painting of a salad. Think about it!"

Proponents of the Paleo Diet differ quite a bit in their dietary prescriptions. Still, they all agree that people today should eat mainly meat, fish, vegetables, and fruit and avoid or limit cereals, legumes and pulses, dairy products, salt, and refined sugar.

The paleo diet has almost 5 thousand articles on [Google Scholar](#).

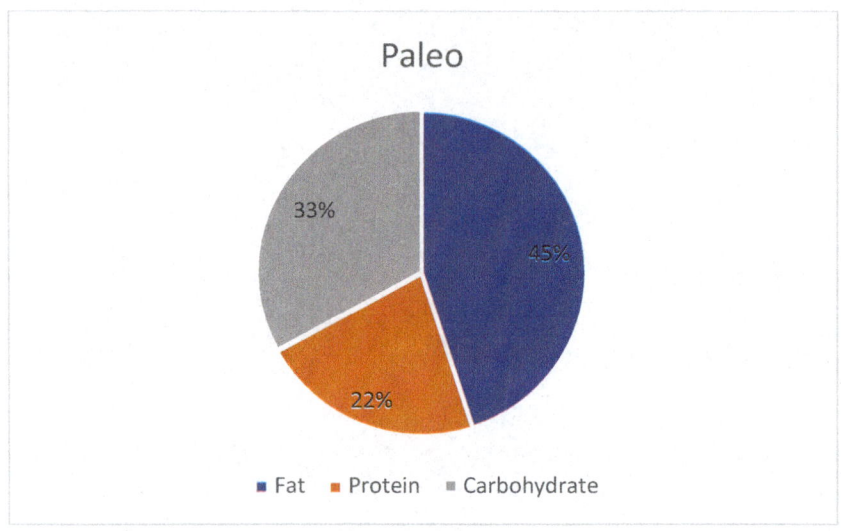

Figure 9 - Macronutrient ratio in the Paleolithic diet

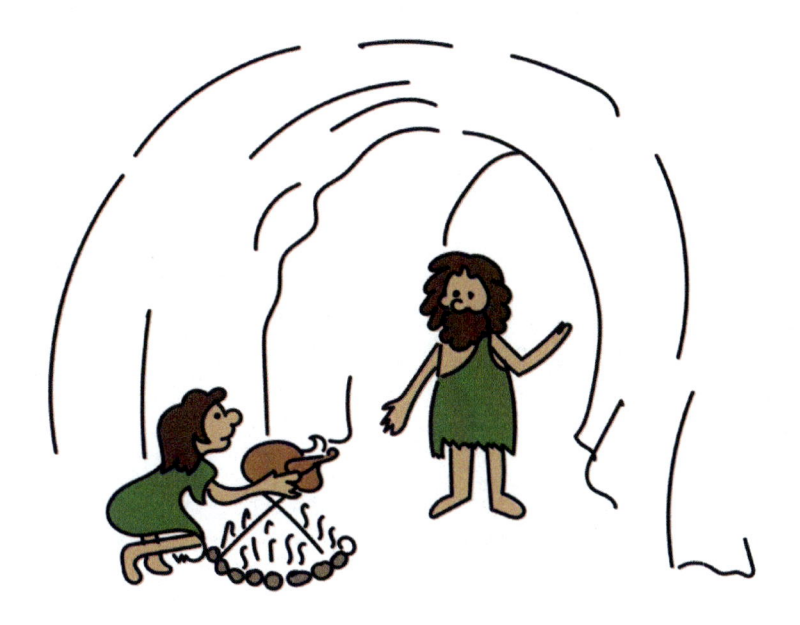

"Don't tell me it's paleo again!"

Mediterranean Diet

The Mediterranean diet is more than a menu for a few days. It is one of the most academically studied diets, with 136 thousand articles on Google Scholar. It is a **lifestyle** and a way of eating based on foods easily found in nature, such as fruits, vegetables, cereals, seeds, fish, and others.

This menu is typical of residents of the Mediterranean region, including the south of countries such as France, Italy, Spain, and Greece. Because of natural nutrition, these people enjoy a longer lifespan, healthier lifestyle, and reduced risk of developing diseases (Figure 10).

The Mediterranean diet's basis is "natural food," free from industrial processing. That is, those foods that can be found in nature and are not packaged, such as fruit, vegetables, fish, eggs, seeds, honey, whole grains, and lean meats. These should be the basis of a menu inspired by a Mediterranean diet. However, it is possible to incorporate other natural foods with minimal processing, such as olive oil, milk, and dairy.

For starters, industrialized foods should be immediately avoided or at least reduced. These items have undergone several production processes, including incorporating unhealthy substances such as dyes and preservatives, and end up losing beneficial food components such as fiber and other nutrients.

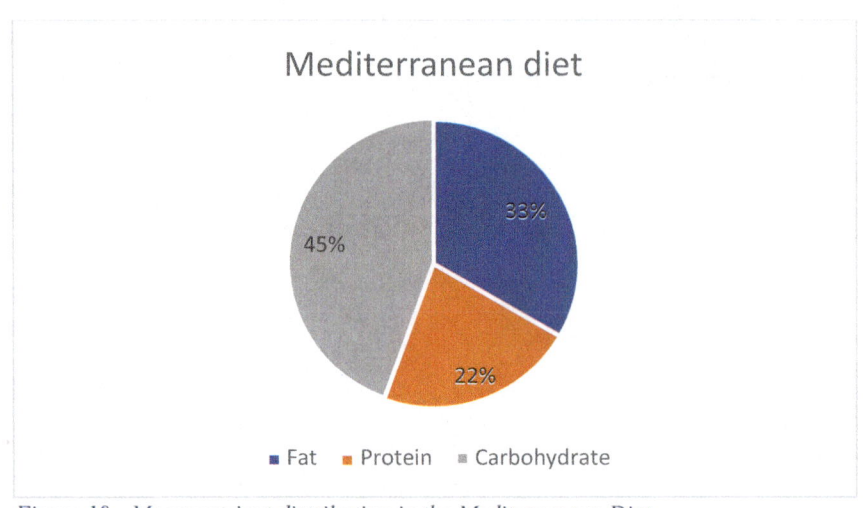

Figure 10 - Macronutrient distribution in the Mediterranean Diet

Intermittent fasting

According to research carried out in 1997, reducing the amount of food available (calorie restriction) during life has beneficial effects on aging and life expectancy in animals[26]. But one thing they failed to remember at the time is that animals on a calorie restriction diet eat everything at once and then go on a 20-hour intermittent fast when ketosis occurs. More recent studies suggest that the benefits of intermittent fasting are not only due to the calorie restriction, which results in weight loss and reduced free radicals, but also because it stimulates cellular response to improve glycemia regulation, increase resistance to stress, and reduce inflammation. During fasting, the liver transforms energy from fatty acids into ketones, and the oxidative defense and molecular repair pathway is activated. During feeding, energy comes from glucose, and cells grow and plasticize. But ketones are not just energy. They are potent signaling molecules that alter cell and organ function, regulating the activity of proteins and molecules that influence health and aging. Serum ketones increase 8 to 12 hours after the start of fasting, reaching high levels of 2 to 5 mmol/L within 24 hours. However, most people in the modern world eat three meals a day, plus snacks. Therefore, natural intermittent fasting does not occur. Natural overnight fasting is not enough to cause a significant increase in ketones in the blood. The three types of intermittent fasting most studied in humans are fasting every other day, fasting 5:2 (fasting two days a week), and fasting daily. This type of fasting consists of not eating solid food for 16 to 36 hours at a time, a few times a week, on a scheduled basis, and returning to the usual diet, preferably based on foods low in sugar and fat. Periods of calorie restriction should, therefore, be planned.

To achieve the benefits, the most common strategy for starting this fast is to go without food for 14 or 16 hours, drinking only liquids such as water, tea, and coffee without sugar. The increase in the fasting period should be gradual. Clinical studies have shown reduced weight and fat tissue comparable to continuous restriction and a significant improvement in cardiovascular risk indicators, systemic inflammation, and oxidative stress.

Did you know that the most extended continuous fast ever recorded was 382 days?[27] In this case, a 27-year-old man weighing 207 kg fasted for 382 days with medical monitoring, vitamin and electrolyte supplementation, and non-caloric liquids, reaching 81 kg and staying close to his final weight for five years. No drugs were used.

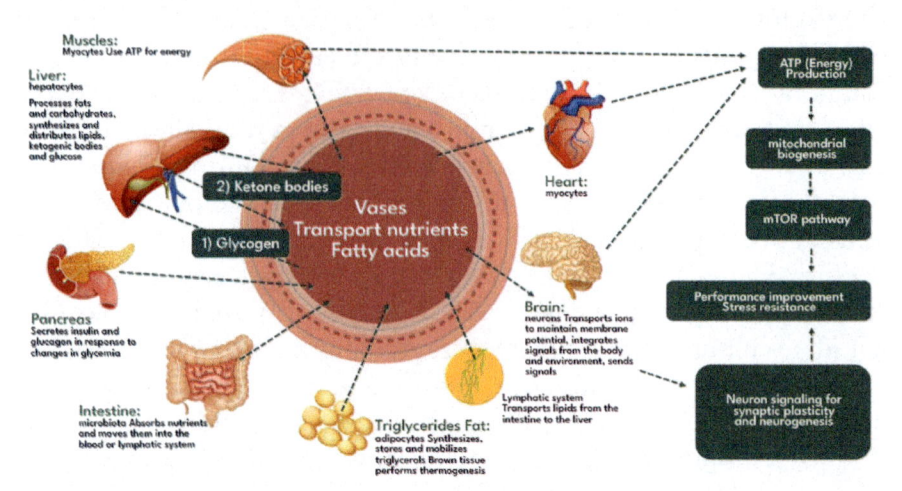

Figure 11 - Metabolic adaptations to intermittent fasting: A *food restriction for 10 to 14 hours depletes liver glycogen and initiates the hydrolysis of triglycerides to fatty acids in adipocytes.* Fatty acids are released into the blood circulation and transported to hepatocytes, producing ketone bodies[26].

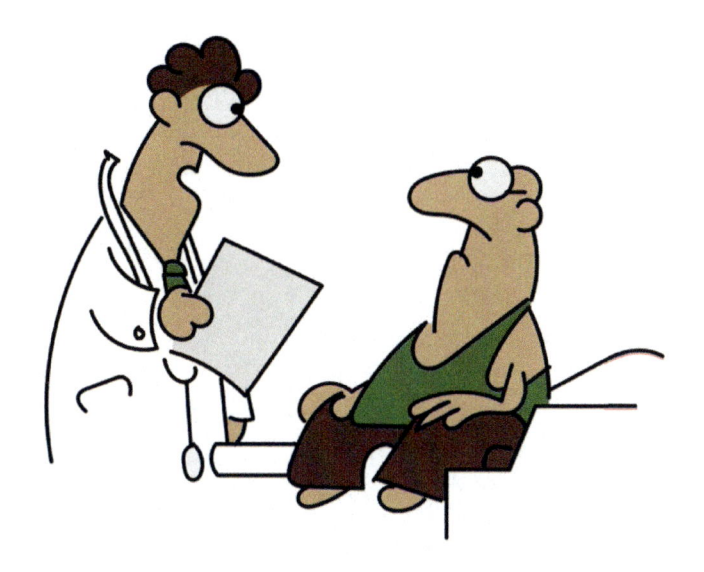

"Your doctor can only do so much, the rest is up to you! Stop getting old"

Commercial ketogenic diets

After the introduction of Dr. Atkins' diet, many have described methodologies for ketogenic diets, such as the South Beach diet and, more recently, the Dukan diet. The Paleolithic diet has been challenged as being a copy of the Dukan diet.

South Beach

The South Beach Diet focuses not only on weight loss but also on a healthy lifestyle. Dr. Arthur Agatston, a physician from Florida, worked in a cardiac prevention center, helping patients control their insulin and cholesterol levels, emphasizing the consumption of good carbohydrates and good fats. The South Beach Diet has almost 2,000 articles on Google Scholar.

The diet starts with an abrupt cut in carbohydrates in the first few weeks, essentially a ketogenic diet, followed by the gradual reintroduction of foods but prioritizing slow-absorbing carbohydrates, i.e., those with a low glycemic index, such as:

- Grains.
- Whole-grain breads and pasta.
- Fruit.
- Beans, soybeans, peas, and lentils.
- Vegetables.

And avoid high-glycemic index carbohydrates as much as possible.

- Sugar.
- Sweets.
- White flour pasta and bread.
- Cassava and potatoes.

Dukan Diet

The Dukan diet, described by Pierre Dukan, was widely accepted by the public but had little academic impact. Like any ketogenic diet, it is based on eating a high amount of protein and a low amount of carbohydrates, but with four different phases and specific rules. It has caused many disputes and disagreements in medical circles, but people love how simple and effective this eating style can be. The Dukan diet has only 300 scientific articles on Google Scholar.

Dukan

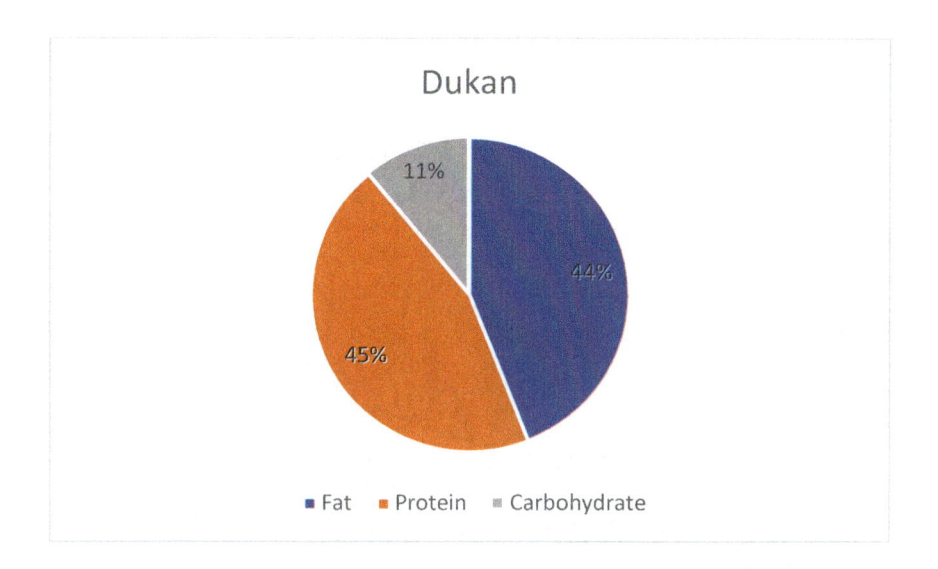

- Fat 44%
- Protein 45%
- Carbohydrate 11%

Harvie and Howell's 2-Day Diet

With their interest in intermittent fasting, Harvie and Howell[28] described the dietary strategies of the two-day diet, with intermittent fasting on two days and a Mediterranean diet on the other days of the week. Often, the days chosen for intermittent fasting are weekdays.

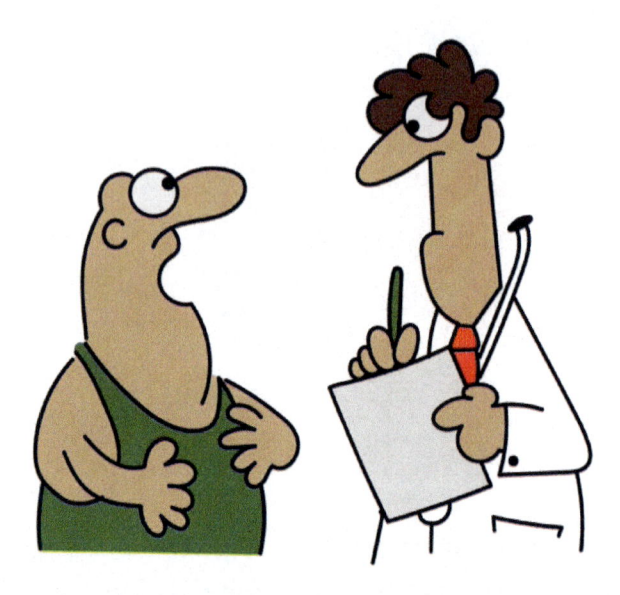

"What's wrong with eating popcorn to lose weight? Don't you believe in alternative medicine?"

Figure 12 - Macronutrient distribution in the fourth phase of the Dukan 28 diet[28]

Important considerations
Effects of the ketogenic diet
The ketogenic diet reduces the amount of glucose circulating in the blood[29] and insulin resistance[29], and can also reduce triglyceride levels[30], increasing HDL (good cholesterol)[29]. The increased satiety induced by ketosis also contributes to weight loss [31].

Gluten

Gluten is a combination of storage proteins called prolamins and glutamins that bind with starch in the endosperm (which feeds the embryonic plant during germination) of the seeds of various cereals of the grass family (*Poaceae*), subfamily *Pooideae*, mainly species of the tribe *Triticeae*, such as wheat, barley, triticale (a hybrid of wheat and rye) and rye. These cereals comprise 40-70% starch, 1-5% lipids, and 7-15% proteins (gliadin, glutenin, albumin, and globulin). Due to its biochemical structure, this type of gluten is often called "triticeae gluten", popularly known as "wheat gluten".

Species of the tribe *Aveneae*, such as oats, do not contain gluten. Still, they are usually processed in factories and mills that also process cereals that have them, thus causing the oats to be contaminated with gluten residues.

Viscosity and elasticity are natural properties of the protein elements in gluten, gliadin (prolamin), and glutenin (glutelin). Gliadin (composed of the sulfur amino acids cystine and cysteine) is a very extensible but inelastic protein responsible for ductility and cohesion. At the same time, glutenin is the polymer responsible for the structure's elasticity. The complex combination of these two long protein chains forms a mass with cohesive and viscoelastic properties in which the gluten retains water in the interstices of the protein chains.

Until recently, it was believed that gluten intolerance was restricted to those with celiac disease and wheat allergy. However, in recent years, several scientific articles have proven that gluten also affects people who don't have these diseases. This new entity has been named non-celiac gluten sensitivity. But it is not that new, as early reports date back three decades. The actual prevalence of non-celiac gluten sensitivity is unknown, as many patients self-diagnose and treat themselves with a gluten-free diet without seeing a doctor. However, estimates suggest it could range between 6% and 63% of the population. The problem appears to be more common in young and middle-aged women.

Symptoms are similar to irritable bowel syndrome, such as abdominal pain, flatulence, bloating, diarrhea, and constipation, in addition to systemic symptoms, such as headache, muscle, and joint pain, chronic fatigue, cramps, limb numbness, brain fog, loss of muscle mass, anemia, eczema, erythema, hyperactivity, ataxia, attention disorder and depression. Symptoms appear hours or days after ingesting gluten.

The diagnosis is made with a food test on a gluten-free diet for three weeks. There is no specific laboratory marker for non-celiac gluten sensitivity. Antigliadin IgG antibody markers occur in only half of patients.

Gluten also causes increased intestinal permeability. When ingested, gluten enters the gastrointestinal tract, and its glutamine and prolamin proteins are partially hydrolyzed by proteases present in the gastrointestinal tract. There is an increase in the peptide zonulin, involving the regulation of cell junctions, which is responsible for the increased intestinal permeability.

Gluten allergy is mediated by IgE antibodies, with ω5-gliadin being the primary allergen.

Gluten-free diet.
There is only one proven method of treating non-celiac gluten sensitivity, which is, of course, the complete removal of gluten from the diet. There is little information on the minimum tolerable amount, which can vary between 10 and 100mg daily. Completely removing all gluten from the diet is not always possible due to contamination in food preparation and trace amounts in foods and drugs.

Gluten-free products are usually made with refined flour and low-fiber starches, necessary for a healthy diet. The gluten-free diet is also associated with vitamin C, B12, D, and folic acid deficiencies. Therefore, eating fruit and taking antioxidants or vitamin supplements is recommended. Folate refers to a natural form of the vitamin, while folic acid refers to the supplement added to food and drink. As wheat flour is fortified in Brazil and is an essential source of iron and folic acid (Vitamin B9), removing this readily available source requires special attention. Foods without gluten, and thus without wheat flour, are low in folate and need to be replaced or adjusted in the diet. The foods naturally richest in folate are dark green vegetables such as parsley, spinach, beet, cabbage, broccoli, cauliflower, and Brussels sprouts, fruits such as avocado, strawberries, and raspberries, and grains such as chickpeas, lentils, and beans. Walnuts and chestnuts, too.

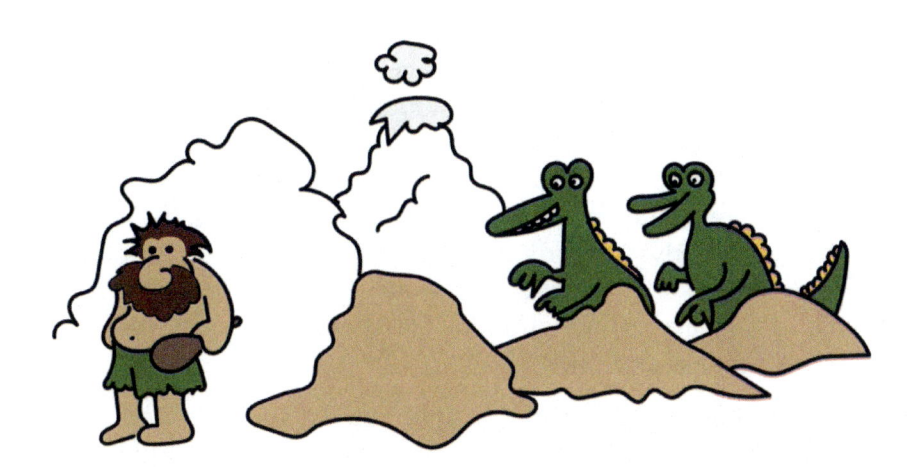

"Not only are they tasty...
they're gluten-free too."

Side effects of the ketogenic diet

Side effects rarely result in diet discontinuation, but they should be observed and reported to the attending physician. Initially, acidosis, hypoglycemia, gastrointestinal events, dehydration, and lethargy may occur. Due to the increased diuresis at the beginning, a significant increase in water intake is recommended.

Hypoglycemia can momentarily cause tremors, paleness, poor motor coordination, poor concentration, headache, dizziness, confusion, hunger, fatigue, fainting, sweating, anxiety, nervousness, and drowsiness. Dehydration causes thirst, dry mouth, dark yellow urine, muscle pain, loss of balance, dizziness, headache, drowsiness, irritability, weakness, and reduced blood pressure. Both can impair judgment and have confounding symptoms. However, hypoglycemia is repeatedly blamed for the symptoms, although dehydration is much more common. When hypoglycemia occurs, it is quickly resolved by the body, which begins the neo-glycogenesis process by recruiting stored energy and increasing glycemia within a few minutes. In the case of dehydration, our organism cannot resolve it without proper rehydration.

These symptoms are typically transient and easily controlled if you are not fasting. But in the long term, the chances of dyslipidemia[xiii], kidney stones (nephrocalcinosis), and stunted growth in children have been suggested. Studies on the changes in the lipid profile are not yet conclusive[32,33]. Some studies show LDL increases, while others show decreases. The increased LDL and cholesterol levels that may occur in some patients are not yet predictable. Despite this, variations are often at near-normal levels. It was also suggested that

---

[xiii]Dyslipidemia (usually hyperlipidemia or hyperlipoproteinemia) is an imbalance in blood lipid and/or lipoprotein levels. Lipids (fatty molecules) are transported in a protein capsule, and the density of the lipids and the type of protein determine the destination of the particle and its influence on metabolism.

increased LDL would not increase cardiovascular risk due to its larger structural size.

Cholesterol and lipids are affected by the diet, with increased both very low-density and low-density lipoproteins that are atherogenic. That is, they form atherosclerotic plaques. It also reduces the amount of antiatherogenic high-density lipoproteins. That is, they reduce the body's natural protection against atherogenesis. In a study of children on a ketogenic diet monitored for two years, cholesterol levels increased by around 130% and stabilized after two years. Lipid lipid levels returned to normal in children over six years old on a ketogenic diet. The long-term effects are not known, but it is known that epileptic children remained on the diet for two years and then returned to their regular diet. Hyperlipidemia is a common effect and can occur in 60% of children on the ketogenic diet, with genetics and the source of dietary fat being the main factors[34]. One study showed that taking 1 to 2g of omega-3 supplements four times daily normalizes the ratio of fatty acids to omega-3 fatty acids [35]. Fenton showed that when hyperlipidemia occurs, dietary choices designed to reduce saturated fats and cholesterol in the diet are enough to normalize the lipid profile[36]. No studies are showing a ketogenic diet as a cardiovascular risk factor[34].

Kidney stones have been reported in studies with epileptic children taking drugs and occur in 5% of children on a ketogenic diet. They are believed to be secondary to acidosis, urinary acidification, hypercalciuria, and hypocitraturia, also triggered by the drugs taken. In these cases, the risk of kidney stones decreased by prophylactic potassium citrate to alkalize the urine[37]. Some antiepileptic drugs have secondary mechanisms of action that can increase the risk of nephrolithiasis, and, in the beginning, some centers even recommended water restriction, which could also contribute to stone formation.

Maintaining bone health is crucial, particularly in assessing the risk of fractures due to osteopenia. In children with epilepsy, the use of antiepileptic drugs can lead to conditions like rickets and osteoporosis. The reason for these conditions is that antiepileptic drugs interfere with vitamin D functionality and calcium absorption and directly impact the processes of bone remodeling[34]. Therefore, vitamin D supplementation and physical exercise are suggested to improve bone health[34]. Periodic monitoring with DEXA[xiv] is optional.

When monitoring younger children being treated for epilepsy, growth can be affected, and bone fractures can occur. Nevertheless, the benefits were more significant than taking antiepileptic drugs, and there are additional factors that can contribute to these events, such as taking certain drugs [38]. Increasing protein and total calories is recommended to avoid stunted growth[34].

Electrolyte and vitamin deficiencies can occur if the diet is not implemented correctly.

The ketogenic diet results in metabolic changes that affect every cell in the body. Many side effects are avoidable with careful monitoring, proper hydration, and diet control. However, some long-term side effects, especially in children, may not be avoidable, and the diet's benefits should constantly be reconsidered.

[xiv]Bone densitometry is a diagnostic method for osteoporosis and osteopenia. It is considered the reference test for measuring bone mineral density. The most commonly used equipment for this examination uses the Dual Energy X-ray Absorptiometry (DEXA) technique.

Ketogenic diet and exercise

There is evidence that diets with more protein allow for more significant muscle gain without increasing body fat. However, recent data shows that low-carb, moderate-protein, and high-fat diets, such as ketogenic diets, can support muscle development and endurance training while promoting fat loss[33]. In the ketogenic diet, there is a glycogen decrease in skeletal muscles and a chronic increase in AMP-activated protein kinase, which has led to the suggestion that it could induce a chronic suppression in the target of rapamycin complex 1 (mTORc1[xv]) in mammals, which leads to protein synthesis, eventually causing stagnation in the anabolic response in resistance training and loss of muscle mass. However, it has been shown in several studies that this undesirable event does not take place[39,40]. Therefore, Physical training is possible with the ketogenic diet as long as adequate hydration is maintained. Many patients on the ketogenic diet notice increased energy during the day [33].

Physical exercise is essential to changing lifestyle habits, as it reduces stress, pain, inflammation, and anxiety and helps maintain and lose weight.

The ketogenic diet increases metabolic flexibility, helping to burn stored fat for energy instead of glucose[41-43]. A study with athletes showed that runners who have adapted to the ketogenic diet can burn 2 to 3 times more fat per minute of exercise compared to low-fat diet runners.

[xv] The mTOR is a central pathway regulating several metabolic processes. Activation of mTORC1 usually culminates in anabolic processes that induce synthesis of proteins, nucleic acids, and lipids

Uses of the ketogenic diet beyond epilepsy

The ketogenic diet is being investigated for various clinical situations. The mechanism of the ketogenic diet in neuroprotection is simple and is also being studied for Parkinson's, Alzheimer's, and astrocytoma[xvi]. In some cases, migraines and narcolepsy can be reduced. There have also been studies into autism, depression, type 2 diabetes, polycystic ovary syndrome, and hypercholesterolemia. The ketogenic diet has also shown benefits as an adjunct in the fight against cancer, especially when detected early[44–47]. The ketogenic diet can help treat obesity, gastroesophageal reflux, diabetes, polycystic ovary, irritable bowel syndrome, non-alcoholic fatty liver disease, post-bariatric weight gain, lymphedema, and lipedema[48].

The ketogenic diet has been shown to treat metabolic syndrome and reduce body weight, BMI, and plasma insulin. It also lowers serum triglycerides and increases HDL (good) without increasing LDL (bad) and creatinine. It also reduces blood pressure, glycemia, and abdominal circumference [49–52].

Lipedema
"Do you feel like there's something wrong with your legs, but you don't know what it is?"

Amato et al.[53]

Lipedema was first described in 1940 by doctors Edgar Van Nuys Allen, a cardiovascular surgeon known for the Allen test, and Edgar Alphonso Hines Jr. at the Mayo Clinic [54,55] in the Vascular Clinics

---

[xvi] Astrocytomas are tumors (neoplasms) of the central nervous system that originate from an astrocyte, a star-shaped cell that supports neurons. This is the most common type of glioma, and they can be benign or malignant. The lower the grade, the longer the survival time, which can exceed 10 years (grade I) or be less than 1 year (grade IV). They affect 5 in every 100,000 people.

section, and today it is named the Allen-Hines syndrome [56]. Since then, lipedema has been characterized as an abnormal bilateral deposition of fat in the buttocks and legs that can be accompanied by orthostatic edema[54,55]. Professor Irany Novah Moraes described *lipophilia* as a preferential distribution of fat to specific body areas in our country. The sexual factor influences this tendency, but with some variations that suggest a certain metamerism. Thus, he proposed five types of preferential fat distribution: *cervicalis*, *humeralis*, *abdominalis*, *membralis,* and *coxalis,* with two subtypes: gluteal or *steatopygial* and *trochanterian* or *cavalarian*[57].

The pathophysiology and epidemiology of lipedema are poorly understood and are therefore not included in the usual academic medical curriculum. So do not expect your doctors to diagnose lipedema quickly, although its signs can be very typical. Lipedema is often confused with more common conditions such as obesity and lymphedema[58,59]. Despite this, recognition of lipedema among the lay public has increased in recent years, partly due to the proliferation of content on the internet and online groups. The beginning of the common media's recognition of this condition and the self-assessment questionnaire published by our research group [53].

Lipedema diagnosis is essentially clinical and is defined by the symmetrical disproportion of fat accumulation in the lower extremities accompanied by complaints of orthostatic edema [58], often accompanied by pain or sensitivity to touch. The feet are spared from this enlargement except in the advanced stage of lipolymphedema when lymphatic insufficiency occurs[60,61]. Swelling that spares the feet is an essential sign for distinguishing lipedema from lymphedema and obesity. The torso is spared. There are cases of lipedema in the upper limbs, in which the fat accumulates in the forearms and arms, sparing the hands, simulating the appearance of fat distribution in the legs[62–65].

Areas affected by lipedema often present bruising, pain, and increased sensitivity accompanied by systemic complaints of fatigue and decreased physical condition and muscle strength. The onset of symptoms occurs during puberty, pregnancy, menopause, or another trigger event[58]. The progression of the disease can occur at critical times of hormonal disturbance, such as pregnancy or the menopause[66]. Lipedema almost exclusively affects women, although it can rarely happen in men[55,58,67]. Conservative estimates of the prevalence of lipedema range from 0.06% to 39% [68,69], and no known ethnic correlation was found. Our prevalence study in Brazil showed 12.3%[70] of women affected, suggesting that 8.8 million adult Brazilian women between the ages of 18 and 69 may suffer from symptoms of lipedema.

In addition, up to 50% of patients with lipedema are overweight or obese, which makes diagnosis difficult. It can be challenging to distinguish between lipedema and other physiological body shapes, as the disproportionate fat distribution typical of lipedema can easily be confused with gynaecoid disproportion, also called pear-shaped obesity[71].

As obesity is defined as a BMI greater than 30 kg/m^2, according to this criterion, many patients with lipedema may end up being classified as obese. This narrow definition of obesity does not consider the fat to lean tissue ratio or even body distribution [58,63]. Unlike common obesity, the fat in lipedema is little influenced by a low-calorie diet or strenuous exercise [64]. In patients with lipedema, targeted treatment for obesity can reduce body volume and weight. Still, the disproportion of the limbs caused by lipedema and the distribution of fat and symptoms can persist. It is, therefore, important to differentiate between the conditions, as the treatment is different, and specific interventions for lipedema are essential to prevent the progression of the disease.

The typical sign of lipedema is classically described as the "tree trunk" or "elephant" legs that get worse as the disease progresses. Subcutaneous fat is deposited above the malleoli, with excess fat settling in a "baggy pants" distribution. The fact that the feet are spared causes a noticeable abrupt change at ankle height between the widened legs and the normal-looking feet, especially in the more advanced stages. This characteristic is known as the fat pad sign[58], "bracelet effect," or even "cuff sign "[71]. In some cases, this cuff can be duplicated on the arms with the wrist[63,64]. A common complaint is swollen limbs that worsen with orthostasis and hot weather[55].

From stages one to four (Figure 13), lipedema is a disease that can be progressive if left untreated, advancing in severity throughout a woman's life[72].

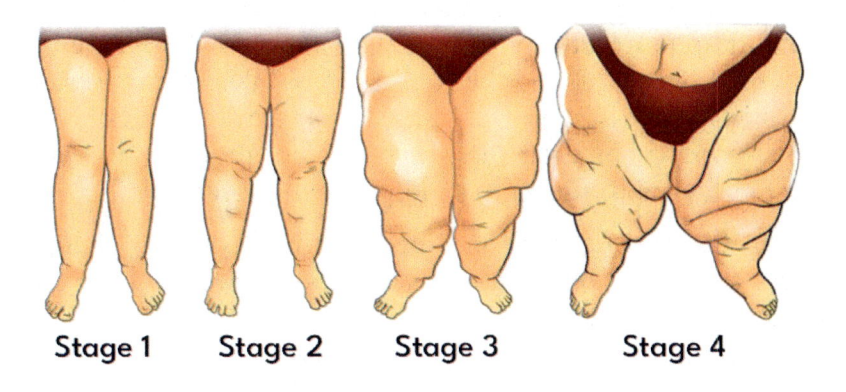

Stage 1   Stage 2   Stage 3   Stage 4

Figure 13 - Lipedema stage classification

Stage I: normal skin with an enlargement of the hypodermis.

Stage II: uneven skin texture with folds of fat and large mounds of tissue growing as unencapsulated masses.

Stage III: hardening and thickening of the subcutaneous tissue with large nodules and protrusion of fat pads, especially on the thighs and around the knees.

Stage IV: lipedema with lymphedema, known as lipolymphedema.

The disease causes progressive discomfort and disfigurement, which invariably leads to psychological and physical suffering.

Another characteristic of lipedema is resistance to obesity treatment. Lipedema fat is resistant to standard diets and non-targeted exercise[58]. In most cases, it is ineffective in reducing weight despite repeated attempts, which may include the inappropriate use of diuretics, a low-calorie diet, regular or even vigorous exercise, compression therapy, or even bariatric surgery [58,73]. When it occurs, weight loss is predominantly in the torso, leaving a persistently lipedemic lower body. The lack of improvement after diet and exercise can also lead to a sense of guilt or failure in patients who are led to believe that they haven't tried hard enough. In a survey conducted in the UK in 2014, a significant number of patients (95%) reported that they failed to lose weight in the areas associated with lipedema despite rigorous measures with substantial improvements and essential results in other body areas [74]. While calorie restriction has proved fruitless, current research into a low-carbohydrate, moderate-protein, high-fat diet has shown promise in weight management, lymphoedema [75,] and lipedema symptoms[4].

The lack of improvement in lipedema with obesity treatment measures has yet to be definitively explained. Still, I believe that while obesity is the cause of inflammation, lipedema is the consequence of inflammation[76]. High rates of malondialdehyde (MDA) and carbonylated proteins, both markers of oxidative stress, i.e., inflammation, have been found in patients with lipedema, including accelerated peroxidation in lipedemic tissue[77]. For this reason, the ketogenic diet can bring significant benefits to some sufferers of this disease, as the ketogenic diet can reduce inflammation.

The evidence keeps adding up. Recently, another case report highlighting the benefits of the long-term ketogenic diet on lipedema was published[78]. The ketogenic diet has a metabolic rationale that induces a reduction in chronic inflammation and regulation of glycemia, avoiding harmful glycemic peaks, but a large-scale study is still lacking.

Ketogenic diet and lipedema
A study (not yet) published but presented by Dr. Faerber from Germany showed that in 100 patients with lipedema, 82.7% of the patients who went on the ketogenic diet improved their lipedema

symptoms, with none showing any worsening, with an average follow-up of 3 years and eight months[79]. Patients felt an improvement in weight and swelling right from the start.

They report improved physical and mental performance. As well as reducing limb volume, the ketogenic diet reduced the need for elastocompression.

The decreased muscle mass in lipedema must be taken into account, and, therefore, the ketogenic diet must be optimized, requiring 1.2 to 1.5g/Kg of protein to preserve muscle. Proteins protect muscle mass and are necessary for the brain, retina, and red blood cells. A practical suggestion is to eat two handfuls of vegetables twice daily so that the required fiber promotes satiety. Less than 50g of carbohydrates per day are allowed to achieve ketosis and beneficial metabolic change. Serum insulin does not increase on diets with less than 35g of carbohydrates per meal and if you don't eat more than 2g of protein per kg of weight. A high amount of fat is necessary if you don't want to lose weight and want to increase ketones.

The ketogenic diet has been shown to have a more significant impact on leptin and insulin levels [xvii]than the low-calorie diet in patients with lipedema[80].

[xvii] Leptin is a peptide that plays an important role in regulating food intake and energy expenditure, generating an increase in energy burning and decreasing food intake. In addition to its well-known effect on appetite control, current evidence shows that leptin is involved in the control of body mass, reproduction, angiogenesis, immunity, healing and cardiovascular function.

Effect of ketones

Insulin[xviii] is the hormone responsible for reducing glycemia by promoting the entry of glucose into cells. It is also essential for carbohydrate metabolism, protein synthesis, and lipid storage. Insulin resistance, also known as insulin resistance, is a condition that precedes many cases of obesity, diabetes, and other metabolic diseases. When an individual has insulin resistance, the body cannot produce the amount of insulin needed to maintain its normal metabolism because the cells require more insulin to act normally, and the pancreas, at a certain point, runs out and cannot produce it. Insulin resistance, therefore, occurs when the action of this hormone, which transports glucose from the blood into the cells, is diminished, even if the amount of insulin in the blood is high, causing glucose to accumulate in the blood, giving rise to metabolic diseases. Insulin resistance is typically pro-inflammatory and, therefore, relevant in lipedema. Insulin prevents lipolysis, i.e., the breakdown of fat into energy. Thus, in insulin resistance, there is an increase in insulin in the blood just when the body needs it most, blocking the breakdown of fat. On the other hand, ketones can maintain low and stable levels of glucose and insulin.

It is theorized that lipedemic adipocytes may require lower insulin levels for lipolysis to occur or that lipedemic adipocytes may be insulin-resistant without systemic insulin resistance. Lipedema indeed manifests itself initially at times of significant hormonal variation in women, which are also phases of systemic insulin resistance, such as adolescence and perimenopause[81]. In general, patients with lipedema have less systemic insulin resistance, but lipedema and obesity are often associated with comorbidities. There is recent evidence of local inflammation in lipedemic adipose tissue, without the traditional inflammatory markers, and in addition, there is the already identified hypertrophy of adipocytes with an increase

---

[xviii]Hormone that regulates the amount of glucose in the blood.

in macrophages[82]. Increased VEGF-C[xix] and inflammatory response are consequences[83].

The ketogenic diet has a diuretic and natriuretic effect; it reduces arachidonic acid levels, reduces aromatase[xx] levels, decreases estradiol[xxi] production in tissues, reduces stress and cortisol, increasing pain tolerance; and Beta-hydroxybutyrate blocks the pro-inflammatory immune reaction[84] by blocking NLRP3[xxii].

As the hormone estradiol increases the sensitivity of adipose tissue to insulin, less insulin is needed to suppress the release of free fatty acids. Fatty tissue in the hip and thigh is sensitive to the action of estrogen[85,86]. Oestradiol appears to decrease pain tolerance. In addition, there is a positive correlation between aromatase activity and an increase in body fat tissue. Insulin stimulates aromatase activity in adipose tissue, thus increasing the distribution of female fat in subcutaneous adipose tissue[87,88]. On the other hand, the interaction between insulin and estradiol reduces pro-inflammatory enzymes (IL1, 6, 8,1 2, TNFα) and, therefore, inflammation. This complex interaction has yet to be better clarified in lipedema.

The ketogenic diet decreases pain[89–91] in lipedema. In 7 weeks, the lowest pain is reached; after six weeks of finishing the diet, the pain returns.

[xix]Vascular endothelial growth factor C is a protein that is a member of the platelet-derived growth factor / vascular endothelial growth factor family.

[xx]Aromatase is an enzyme of the cytochrome P450 group that catalyzes the aromatization of androgens into estrogens, namely the conversion of testosterone into estradiol and androstenedione into estrone.

[xxi]Estradiol or 17β-estradiol is a sex hormone and steroid, the main female sex hormone. It is important in regulating the estrous cycle and the menstrual cycle. Oestradiol is essential for the development and maintenance of female reproductive tissues, but it also has important effects on many other tissues. The hormone oestradiol is also produced in adipose tissue.

[xxii]NLRP3 is a protein that, in humans, is expressed in macrophages as a component of the inflammatory cascade. The inflammasome is an oligomeric protein complex involved in the innate immune system formed after the recognition of various inflammatory signals (LPS, uric acid crystals and various viral and bacterial compounds) by proteins of the NPLR family.

In general, it has been observed that the hormone leptin signals satiety, but in obesity, the brain becomes insensitive or resistant to leptin. Obesity is a disease of resistances: insulin resistance and leptin resistance. The ketogenic diet improves central sensitivity to leptin, increasing satiety, which can be helpful in obesity and lipedema[4].

In the absence of major dietary studies on lipedema, following anecdotal reports from patients and the follow-up of hundreds of patients in an outpatient clinic dedicated to lipedema, we believe the ketogenic diet is an essential tool in controlling lipedema.

The ketogenic diet can impact weight reduction, fat deposition, pain reduction, and improved quality of life. It also suggests that there may be an improvement in metabolism and hormonal function, a reduction in edema and inflammation, and the prevention and reduction of fibrosis.

The ketogenic diet is effective in rapid weight loss, primarily by lowering insulin and increasing satiety with fat intake. The change in cellular energy source from glucose to fat provides a sustainable fat-busting environment without the risk of lean mass loss that occurs with low-calorie diets[4].

There are a few explanations for why the ketogenic diet allows the loss of adipose tissue in lipedema. In contrast, other diets do not: lipedemic adipocytes may need lower insulin levels for lipolysis to occur, have impaired sensitivity to glucagon[xxiii], and/or be insulin resistant despite systemic insulin sensitivity. This last possibility is the most promising. Keith suggests that the onset of lipedema occurs at times of systemic insulin resistance and that hypertrophied adipocytes are linked to insulin resistance[4].

The ketogenic diet decreases adipocyte size, insulin levels, and serum leptin. Higher insulin levels promote lipogenesis and

---

[xxiii] Glucagon is a hormone (polypeptide) produced in the pancreas and in the cells of the gastrointestinal tract that is important in carbohydrate metabolism. Its best-known role is to increase glycemia by counteracting the effects of insulin.

adipocyte hypertrophy. These aspects are essential when considering the treatment of lipedema. Keith also suggests that the metabolic changes induced by ketosis control adipocyte proliferation and inflammation in lipedema in three ways: by reducing adiposity through lipolysis for energy, by decreasing insulin to levels low enough to allow lipolysis of lipedemic adipocytes, by suppressing appetite by increasing glucagon and by preventing the progression of the disease. Glucagon works oppositely to insulin, a catabolic hormone that controls hypoglycemia and is involved in energy homeostasis and the metabolism of lipids and amino acids, as well as an essential stress hormone. In short, glucagon increases satiety, decreases food intake, and increases energy expenditure and heat production. Glucagon resistance may contribute to the deposition of fatty tissue, lower temperature, and reduced satiety found despite the low prevalence of insulin resistance and type 2 diabetes in patients with lipedema.

The ketogenic diet can decrease lipedemic pain probably because the mechanisms of pain and inflammation are shared, and the ketosis induced by the ketogenic diet decreases the excitability of neurons, which, in a way, can suppress the perception of pain, block glycolysis, reduce inflammation and increase the levels of adenosine, a natural analgesic. In addition, carbohydrate diets are associated with a higher incidence of anxiety and depression, which are not exclusive to patients with lipedema but can be treated and help clinical improvement by removing carbohydrates from the diet.

The ketogenic diet can also reduce the sensation of water retention without the use of diuretics, which worsens lipedema. Interestingly, it has also been shown in rats that ketone bodies can activate lymphangiogenesis, i.e., the growth and development of new lymphatic vessels, something previously thought impossible[15].

Decreased inflammation with the ketogenic diet has been shown in some studies. Ketone bodies modulate inflammation and reduce oxidative stress. The results of a randomized controlled study of overweight men and women comparing the ketogenic diet and the low-fat diet suggest that the composition of macronutrients and not calorie restriction or weight loss produces the most outstanding anti-inflammatory effects. It is important to remember that we recommend a strategic anti-inflammatory diet[xxiv] as the first line of treatment for lipedema. The ketogenic diet, which is also anti-inflammatory, is one of the therapeutic options. My strategy in initially choosing the anti-inflammatory diet is because some people can have inflammatory reactions to foods that are present in the ketogenic diet, among the most frequent being milk, cheese, and eggs. Therefore, this self-knowledge is necessary before starting a ketogenic diet.

Little is currently known about the fibrosis caused by lipedema, but it has been shown that the ketogenic diet can reduce fibrosis in fibrotic livers with non-alcoholic disease[92–94].

The improvement in clinical symptoms is evident with weight reduction and metabolism normalization. Remember that lipedema is not treated with diet alone but with lifestyle changes and, in some selected cases, appropriate surgery.

[xxiv]Book: Strategic Anti-Inflammatory Diet. Dr. Alexandre Campos Moraes Amato. https://bio.amato.io/livro

The ketogenic diet for weight loss

Obesity is one of the most common medical problems and a significant risk factor in cardiovascular disease, along with dyslipidemia, hypertension, and diabetes, which make up the metabolic syndrome.[95]

Various strategies have been proposed, with the basic principle being to reduce intake and increase energy expenditure. Regarding dieting, there are many conflicting opinions and different types and proposals for weight loss. The most commonly accepted principle, probably because of its inherent simplicity, is to reduce calorie intake, often by reducing fat intake.

Despite the proven usefulness of the ketogenic diet in various pathological situations, it is most often used for weight loss. And when done correctly, it works. Undoubtedly, the ketogenic diet is very effective in the short and medium term in fighting obesity and hyperlipidemia and improving metabolism and cardiovascular risk factors, as demonstrated above. Despite its effectiveness, its complex and obscure mechanism raises concerns. As scientific studies on diets are not easy to carry out because the double-blind, randomized approach is not possible, some answers may not have sufficient evidence to satisfy the most critical. Undeniably, the principle of the ketogenic diet, physiological ketosis, changes the body's metabolism. More and more evidence shows the beneficial effects of ketone bodies and these metabolic changes, but only time will cement this knowledge. "Insanity is doing the same thing repeatedly and expecting different results," said Albert Einstein. Curiously, even after several previous therapeutic failures, many still prefer to insist on the strategies adopted previously rather than experience the radical metabolic change induced by ketosis.

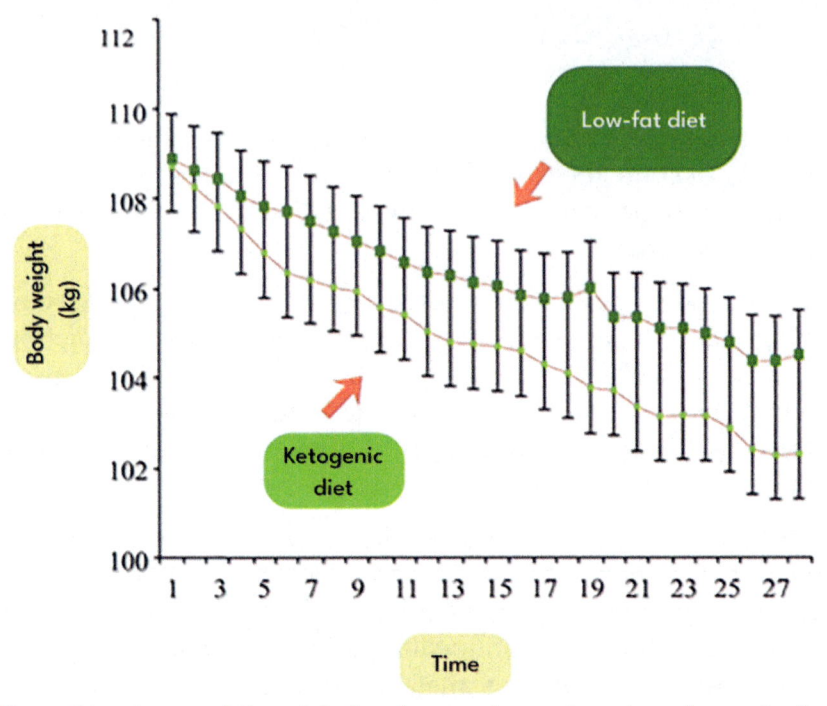

Figure 14 - Average daily weight loss between ketogenic and non-ketogenic diet with minimal difference in calories[28]

It is obvious today that abdominal obesity is a risk factor for metabolic diseases[96,97], and may increase the risk of cardiovascular disease and type 2 diabetes, as well as premature death. But few remember that lower limb fat has been suggested to have a protective effect on cardiovascular risk in women[98]. The ketogenic diet effectively reduces abdominal fat and, consequently, cardiovascular risk.

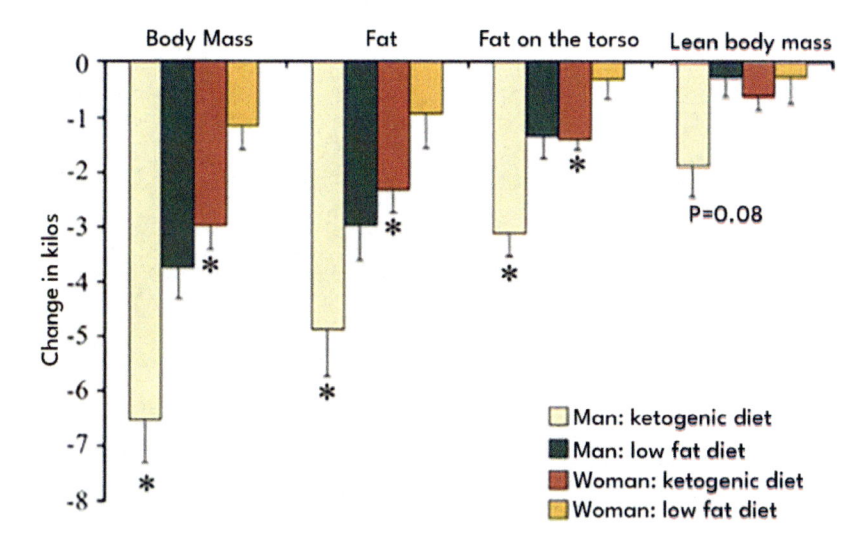

Figure 15 - Comparison of fat loss among diets[97]

Physiology of ketosis

We will get a little more technical in this chapter. If you're not interested in the biology behind the diet, skip this chapter.

After a few days of fasting or a drastic decrease in carbohydrates in the diet (below 20g per day), the body's glucose reserve becomes insufficient to produce oxaloacetate for the normal oxidation of fat in the Krebs cycle and to supply glucose to the central nervous system.

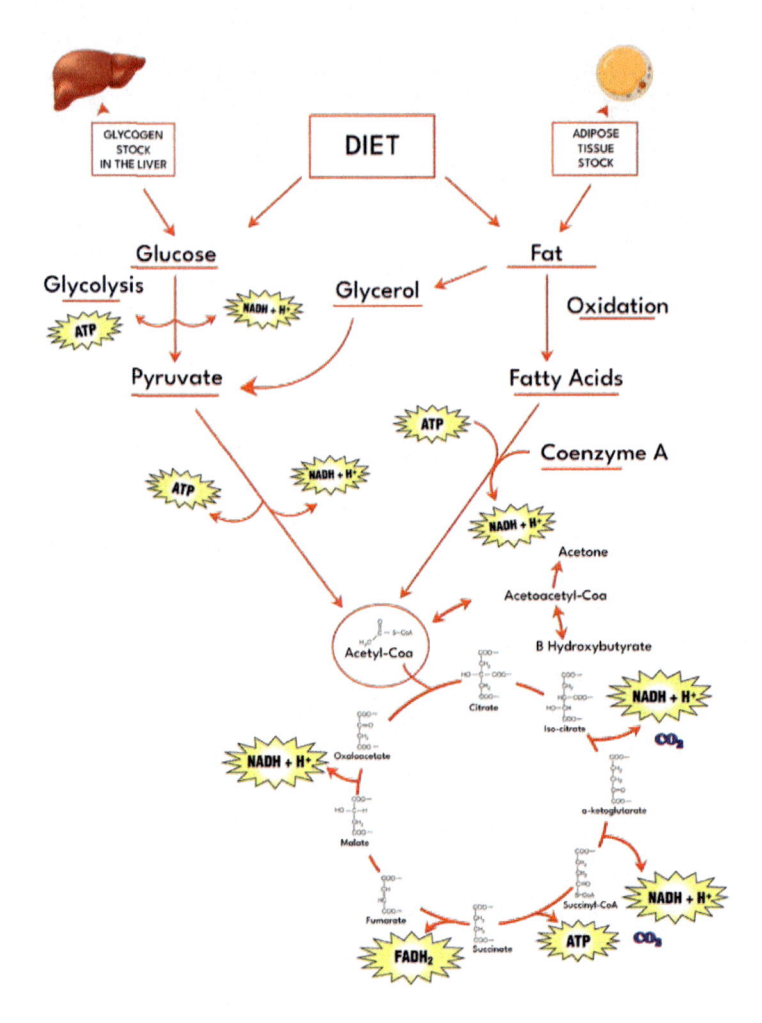

Figure 16 - Krebs Cycle: The Krebs Cycle, also known as the Tricarboxylic Acid Cycle and the Citric Acid Cycle, refers to a series of anabolic and catabolic reactions to produce energy for cells. This is one of the three stages of the cellular respiration process.

Oxalacetate is relatively unstable at body temperature, so it is necessary to supply the tricarboxylic acid cycle with glucose-derived oxaloacetate through ATP-dependent carboxylation of pyruvic acid by pyruvate carboxylase.

The central nervous system can't use fatty acids as an energy source because they don't pass the blood-brain barrier, so glucose is the only fuel for the human brain.

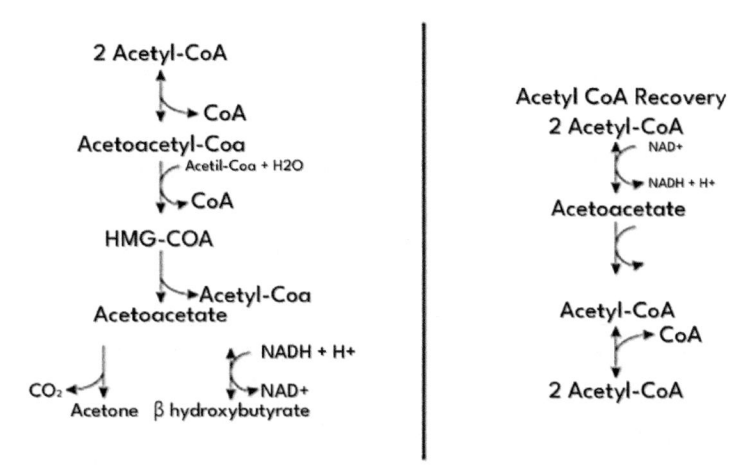

Figure 17 - Ketone bodies: The acetyl-CoA formed by the beta-oxidation steps can go to various destinations, and its use in the Krebs Cycle is of central importance. An alternative pathway is the synthesis of ketone bodies, which occurs in the mitochondrial matrix and is primarily a liver function since the enzyme HMG-CoA synthase is present in large quantities only in this tissue. The acetoacetate and beta-hydroxybutyrate, thus produced (the formation of acetone is usually less important), are transported by the blood to other tissues, where they are reconverted to acetyl-CoA. The enzyme b-oxyacid-CoA transferase is present in all tissues except the liver. This ensures that reconversion to acetyl-CoA only occurs in extrahepatic tissues, thus avoiding a futile cycle. Both are mitochondrial enzymes. This is an essential source of energy for some cells during prolonged fasting. These include nerve cells, which do not have the cellular apparatus to use lipids as an energy source (they do not carry out beta-oxidation). Thus, in the absence of glucose, they only have this source of acetyl-CoA to use in the Krebs Cycle. Red blood cells also depend on glucose but cannot use ketone bodies, as they do not have mitochondria.

After 3 to 4 days of fasting or low carbohydrate intake, the central nervous system needs an alternative energy source, and it finds it in the overproduction of acetyl-coenzyme-A (Acetyl-CoA), which leads to the production of ketone bodies: acetoacetate, ß-hydroxybutyric acid, and acetone. This process is called ketogenesis and occurs in the mitochondrial matrix in the liver. The liver produces ketone bodies but cannot utilize them due to the absence of the enzyme 3-ketoacylcoenzyme-A transferase, which is needed to convert acetoacetate into acetoacetyl coenzyme A.

Ketone bodies can be used as energy[25], and acetoacetate is the primary ketone body. It is produced and used during metabolism, and other ketone bodies are derived from it. Acetone is produced spontaneously by the decarboxylation of acetoacetate and is important from a clinical point of view as it is responsible for the odor of ketoacidosis. the reduction of acetoacetate produces ß-hydroxybutyric acid.

Although the primary ketone body is acetoacetate, ß-hydroxybutyrate is the main circulating. Under normal conditions, the production of free acetoacetic acid is negligible, and the little that is transported by the blood is metabolized in the muscle tissues. In a situation of increased production of acetoacetic acid, it accumulates at higher than normal levels, and part is converted into other ketone bodies. The presence of ketone bodies in the blood and their elimination in the urine causes ketonuria[xxv] and ketonemia[xxvi]. Acetone, produced by the decarboxylation of acetoacetate, is very volatile and is eliminated in the breath, making a characteristic odor. Acetone has no metabolic use, but its presence serves to diagnose the moment and situation of the diet, and ketogenic breath indicates the condition of ketosis. It can be physiological in a fast, after exercise, or ketogenic diet, and not necessarily due to the disease.

Ketosis is a standard and characteristic state of human metabolism. We are more susceptible to inducing ketosis due to our higher brain/body mass ratio. Under normal conditions, the concentration of ketone bodies is very low (<0.3mmkl/L) compared to glucose (approximately 4mmol) and, with glucose and ketone bodies having a similar Km (Michaelis-Menten constant[xxvii]) in the transport of glucose to the brain, ketone bodies begin to be used as an energy source when the cerebral nervous system reaches a concentration of

---

[xxv] Ketonuria is the presence of ketone bodies in the urine, serving as a sign of decompensation of diabetes mellitus, urinary infection in pregnant women.

[xxvi] Ketosis or ketonemia is a condition characterized by an increase in the concentration of ketone bodies in body fluids (blood, urine, milk and saliva).

[xxvii] In biochemistry, Michaelis-Menten kinetics is one of the best-known models of enzyme kinetics.

4mmol/L, which is close to the Km for the monocarboxylate transporter.

Ketone bodies are used as an energy source through a pathway that involves ß-hydroxybutyric acid converted to acetoacetate and then transformed into acetoacetyl coenzyme-A and, finally, two molecules of acetyl coenzyme-A are formed from acetoacetyl coenzyme-A which are used in the Krebs cycle. Even though glycemia decreases, it remains at physiological levels. Glucose is created through two pathways: amino glucogenic acid and glycerol released by the breakdown of triglycerides. The importance of the second pathway increases progressively with ketosis. In the first days of the ketogenic diet, the main route of glucose formation is the neoglucogenesis of amino acids, and as the days go by, the energy contribution of amino acids decreases, and the amount of glucose derived from glycerol increases. Glycerol, produced by the hydrolysis of triglycerides, can initially produce more than 16% of hepatic glucose during the ketogenic diet and later up to 60%. Of the new glucose formed, 38% comes from glycerol in lean people and 79% in obese people[52].

Table 2 Serum comparison between regular diet, ketogenic diet, and diabetic ketoacidosis

Serum levels	Normal diet	Ketogenic diet	Diabetic ketoacidosis
Glucose (mg/dL)	80-120	65-80	>300
Insulin (µU/L)	6-23	6.6-9.4	0
Ketone bodies (mmol/L)	0.1	7/8	>25
pH	7.4	7.4	<7.3

During physiological ketosis, ketonemia reaches levels of 7 to 8 mmol/L with no change in pH, while in diabetic ketoacidosis, it can exceed 20 mmol/L with a drop in blood pH. In healthy people, ketone bodies do not exceed eight mmol/L because the central nervous system uses these energy molecules efficiently.

Does the ketogenic diet work?

There is no doubt that the ketogenic diet is effective in weight loss. However, the exact mechanism of the diet's effects is still being debated. Atkins' original hypothesis suggested that weight loss was induced by losing energy through the excretion of ketone bodies, but many other theories have been put forward. One is that using protein-derived energy in the ketogenic diet is an expensive metabolic process for the body, leading to a loss of calories and, therefore, more significant weight loss compared to other diets. During the first phase of the ketogenic diet, the body needs 60 to 65g of glucose a day, 16% of which is obtained from glycerol and the rest from protein gluconeogenesis, either from the diet or from the body's own tissue. Gluconeogenesis is a process that requires energy to function, and it is calculated at around 400 to 600 Kcal/day. There is also a decrease in appetite due to the greater satiety of proteins, and the authors also cite a hormonal effect on appetite. Other authors suggest that ketone bodies are appetite suppressants and central satiety signals in their own right. Over time, the improvement in fat oxidation shown by the decrease in respiratory rate may explain the weight and fat loss from this diet.

1. Reduced appetite:
    a. greater satiety from proteins;
    b. appetite hormone control;
    c. direct appetite-suppressing effect of ketone bodies.
2. Reduced lipogenesis and increased lipolysis.
3. Increased metabolic efficiency.
4. Increased energy is required for the metabolic process of neoglycogenesis and the thermal effect of proteins.

Other benefits in obesity

It has been suggested that ketones have a protective effect against the loss of cognition caused by weight gain and obesity. There is evidence that ketogenic diets have a positive effect on mood in overweight patients.

At the beginning of the ketogenic diet, the first 4-5 days, there is a feeling of lethargy, but this effect wears off quickly, and the mood improves afterward.

Insulin resistance is common in obesity, and the fundamental problem lies in carbohydrate metabolism. Therefore, the low-carbohydrate ketogenic diet improves glycemic control, hemoglobin A1c, and lipid markers and reduces the need for exogenous insulin.

Another beneficial effect is increased longevity. Although studies are restricted to animals, the ketogenic diet has had positive effects on metabolic syndrome and cancer risk.

The yo-yo or accordion effect

Several studies have made it clear that the ketogenic diet, in the short term, results in more significant weight loss than other low-fat diets. However, successful treatment is considered to be sustained weight loss over the long term. There are fewer jobs with longer follow-ups. For this reason, some skeptics cite the yo-yo effect as evidence of only transient beneficial effects. The criteria for defining successful weight loss need to be established: individuals who have lost at least 10% of their body weight and maintained it for at least one year. It has been shown that two periods of a ketogenic diet separated by long periods of a Mediterranean diet lead to persistent weight loss and improved risk factors.

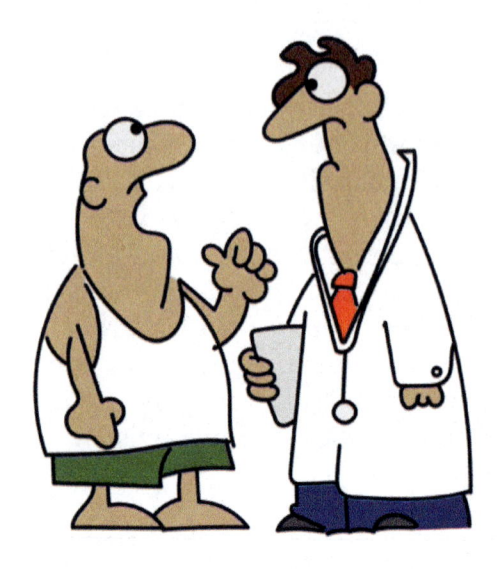

"I could be a healthy person if you'd stop finding things wrong with me!"

Is the ketogenic diet safe?

The first question is always about the increase in lipids. Common sense suggests that a low-carbohydrate, high-protein, high-fat diet cannot be healthy, as it can increase bad cholesterol and triglycerides, which are often a problem in obese people. The first studies, published in the 1950s, showed that increased fat consumption was associated with a higher prevalence of atherosclerosis[99]. Thus, the first recommendation regarding the consumption of fats established a limit of 30% of the total caloric value of the diet in the form of fats and recommended a reduction in the consumption of saturated fatty acids. Despite this, much modern evidence suggests that the ketogenic diet is beneficial in controlling cardiovascular risk factors. The Brazilian Society of Cardiology recognizes that the dietary pattern in which fats are consumed should be taken into account, as they are more harmful when associated with a diet high in sugars and low in fiber, whereas, in a healthy dietary pattern, their negative impact is lower[100].

Most studies show that reducing carbohydrates significantly reduces total cholesterol, increases HDL (good cholesterol), and lowers triglycerides. It also increases the volume of LDL-C particles, which are considered healthier.

There is a biochemical explanation for the synthesis of endogenous cholesterol: the key enzyme in the biosynthesis of cholesterol, HMG-CoA reductase (the target of statins), which is activated by insulin, means that when blood glucose rises, insulin increases and leads to an increase in cholesterol synthesis. Therefore, reducing carbohydrates and an adequate cholesterol intake will lead to an inhibition of cholesterol biosynthesis.

Another common concern is the potentially damaging effect on the kidneys. It is believed that the high levels of nitrogen excretion from protein metabolism can cause an increase in glomerular pressure and hyperfiltration. In patients with intact kidney function, increased protein intake causes morphological and functional adaptations but without adverse effects. We should also consider blood pressure, as kidney function can impact pressure. Amino acids involved in gluconeogenesis and urea production have the effect of lowering blood pressure, while amino acids tend to increase it. Patients with renal insufficiency, even if subclinical, transplant patients, and those with metabolic syndrome or other obesity-related conditions may be more susceptible to the hypertensive effects of amino acids. There is a correlation between obesity and a decrease in the number of nephrons in patients with high blood pressure, and they may be at greater risk. Other studies have shown an improvement in diabetic nephropathy in rats on a ketogenic diet. Some authors have demonstrated the benefit of reducing protein intake from 1.2 g/Kg to 0.9 g/Kg in the short term for type 2 diabetic patients with albuminuria without any long-term benefit. But the proper ketogenic diet isn't hyperproteic; it's normal in protein, with 1.2 to 1.5g of protein per kg of weight.

Concerning possible acidosis, as the concentration of ketone bodies never rises above eight mmol/L, this risk does not exist in those whose insulin functions normally. One common fear is the formation of kidney stones. A study of 195 children on the ketogenic diet showed that 6.7% developed kidney lithiasis[37], but using potassium citrate, an oral alkalizing agent, significantly reduced stone formation. We suggest prophylactic use for those with risk factors, as vigorous hydration seems to be very important in reducing the risk.

Another aspect that should be considered is the effect on bone metabolism. Evidence suggests that a short-term ketogenic diet can impact bone density and the mechanical properties of bones in rats. In humans, it has been shown in children on a ketogenic diet for long periods that there may be a reduction in bone mineral content. On the other hand, obesity, type 2 diabetes, metabolic syndrome, glucose intolerance, insulin resistance, hyperglycemia, and inflammation are associated with an increased risk of fractures.

A period of low-carbohydrate ketogenic dieting can help control hunger, improve oxidative metabolism of fats, and reduce body weight.

Nowadays, some foods that mimic carbohydrates can make it easier to stick to the diet.

Renal function should be assessed during the transition between the ketogenic and regular diets, which should be gradual and controlled.

The duration of the ketogenic diet can vary from a few days (2 to 3 weeks) to induce physiological ketosis to a maximum of several months (6 to 12 months).

It's essential to clarify that the ketogenic diet works for everyone. All human beings can extract energy from fat as long as it is done correctly.

It is essential to follow up with your doctor, as it is often necessary to withdraw medications that are no longer needed.

Hypotheses on the mechanism of action of the ketogenic diet

The pH hypothesis
Proposed in 1931 by Bridge and Iob[101], it suggests that the ketogenic diet makes the blood slightly more acidic and that this influences epileptic episodes. It is based on the fact that fats are used as the primary energy source. The liver ends up metabolizing ketone bodies, acetoacetate, and ß-hydroxybutyric ketoacids. However, it was later proven that diet does not change blood pH.

Metabolic hypotheses
Regarding increased brain energy, DeVivo[102] proposed that ketone bodies are a more efficient energy source than glucose, as they produce more ATP per unit. This would mean that the brain would have more energy available. But glucose continues to exist in the bloodstream, even after weeks of a ketogenic diet.

Concerning the increased mitochondria count, Bough[103,104] suggests that, as in rats, the ketogenic diet produces more mitochondria, which would mean more energy for the brain, adding to the previous hypothesis.

Another theory is that glucose provides quick energy and would prevent seizures in the absence of glucose. Ketone bodies do not produce rapid energy through glycolysis; they must go through the complete Krebs cycle.

Regarding the amino acid theory, ketone bodies would modify the balance of neurotransmitters, suppressing seizures. It suggests that the ketogenic diet increases GABAergic inhibition.

Regarding the ketone theory, ketone bodies would have an anticonvulsant effect by themselves.

Healthy fats

Fat is a macronutrient, also called lipid, found in many food groups. It is the nutrient that has the most kilocalories (9kcal per gram), making it the most caloric. These can be fatty acids, cholesterol, or phospholipids. Fatty acids are the basic structural units of different fats. Essential fatty acids are fats the body cannot produce and must be obtained through food.

The Functions of Fats

Fats are essential for the proper functioning of the human body. They have an energetic function and constitute a reservoir of fuel that the body can use in case of deprivation or the ketogenic diet. It provides internal (organs) and external (impact) body protection, also having a thermal function, in colder regions. The body uses it to constitution cell walls and hormones and protect the nervous system. The brain is an organ with a high percentage of fat. Lipids are one of the brain's main constituents, revealing their importance in human nutrition!

Fat also adds flavor and aroma to food, especially after cooking. It provides a feeling of satiety and can influence the time and quality of digestion and food absorption. Allows better absorption of some vitamins, such as vitamins A, D, E, and K, which are fat-soluble, carried by fats, with functions associated with the renewal and quality of tissues and hormones.

Different fats

Different types of foods provide different amounts and types of fats. There are foods composed almost exclusively of fat, such as olive oil, butter, lard, and oils. Other foods, in addition to fat, also contain proteins, such as meat, eggs, fish, oilseeds, and seeds. Milk, yogurt, and cheese have carbohydrates in addition to fats.

There are, therefore, different types of fats. Saturated and unsaturated fat (monounsaturated and polyunsaturated) have critical bodily functions.

Saturated fat

Saturated fat is found mainly in products of animal origin, such as meat and derivatives, eggs, milk, cheese, yogurt, butter, and cream. Fish contain less of this fat than other meats. Furthermore, fish, especially salmon, sardines, trout, and tuna, have a high omega-3 and alpha-linolenic acid content, which are not synthesized by the human body.

Plant-based foods include coconut and palm oils, which also contain saturated fat.

Grass-fed cattle are generally slaughtered at lower weights than those kept in feedlots, producing leaner total carcasses. These carcasses have the advantage of having a lower total lipid percentage and a higher proportion of favorable unsaturated fatty acids[105]. Thus, saturated fats from pasture-raised animals have a softer impact on cardiovascular risk, so prefer fat from pasture-raised animals.

Mono and polyunsaturated fats

Mono and polyunsaturated fats are known for their beneficial effects on health:

In the group of monounsaturated fats, there is oleic acid, also called omega 9.

It is used for structural functions such as cell membranes and is present in tissues such as the epidermis, contributing to the protection and prevention of dehydration. It is in olive oil, olives, avocados, nuts, and peanut oil.

Polyunsaturated fat contains linoleic acid, also called omega 6.

This, if consumed in large portions, can have a pro-inflammatory behavior. For this reason, and because it is found in foods with considerable caloric content, consumption shouldn't be very high in quantity. You can find it in soybean, corn, sunflower, and linseed oil.

Several foods contain both types, omega six and omega 3, in different amounts.

Omega 3 fatty acids, such as alpha-linolenic acid (ALA), eicosapentaenoic acid (EPA), and docosahexaenoic acid (DHA), help in the development and reasonable maintenance of the central nervous system and vision. They have more potent anti-inflammatory properties than omega-6.

Its consumption contributes to lowering the risk of cardiovascular disease and reducing LDL (low-density lipoprotein, known as bad cholesterol — in excess, it is deposited in the blood vessels and can lead to atherosclerosis), triglycerides, and increasing HDL (high-density lipoprotein, also known as good cholesterol), as well as lowering blood pressure.

Some fish are made up of more of these fatty acids. This is the case with mackerel, salmon, sardines, tuna, and seaweed. Oilseeds (such as walnuts) and seeds (such as flaxseed) are also rich in these components.

In short, saturated and unsaturated fats have essential and distinct properties and play an important role in health as long as they are consumed in moderation so as not to do more harm than good, especially in cardiovascular health.

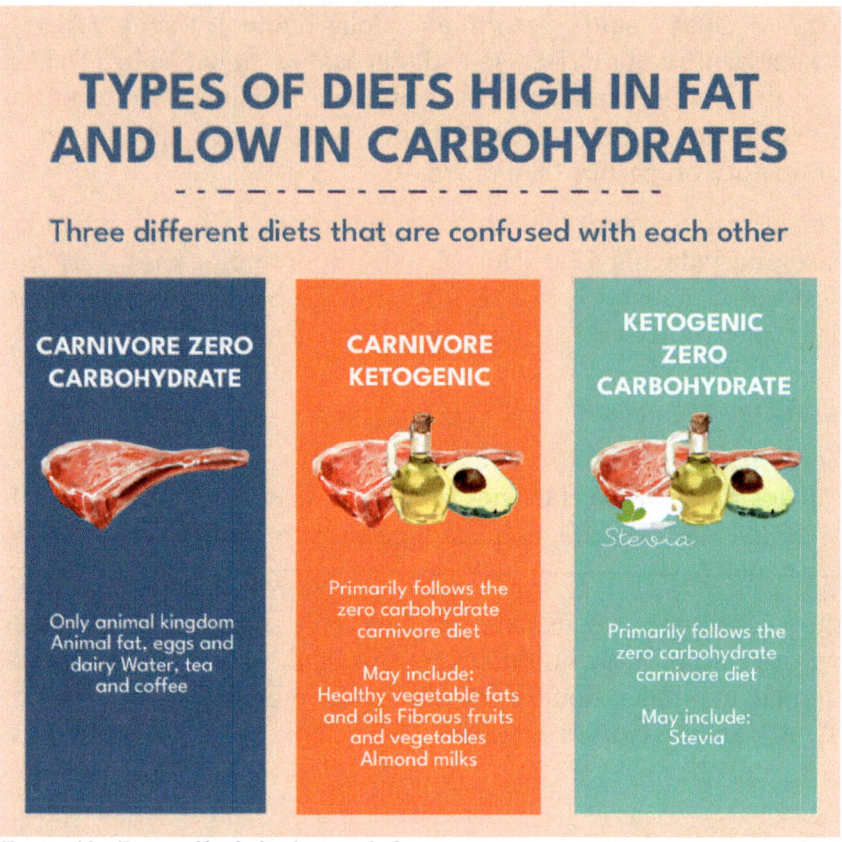

Figure 18 - Types of high-fat, low-carb diets

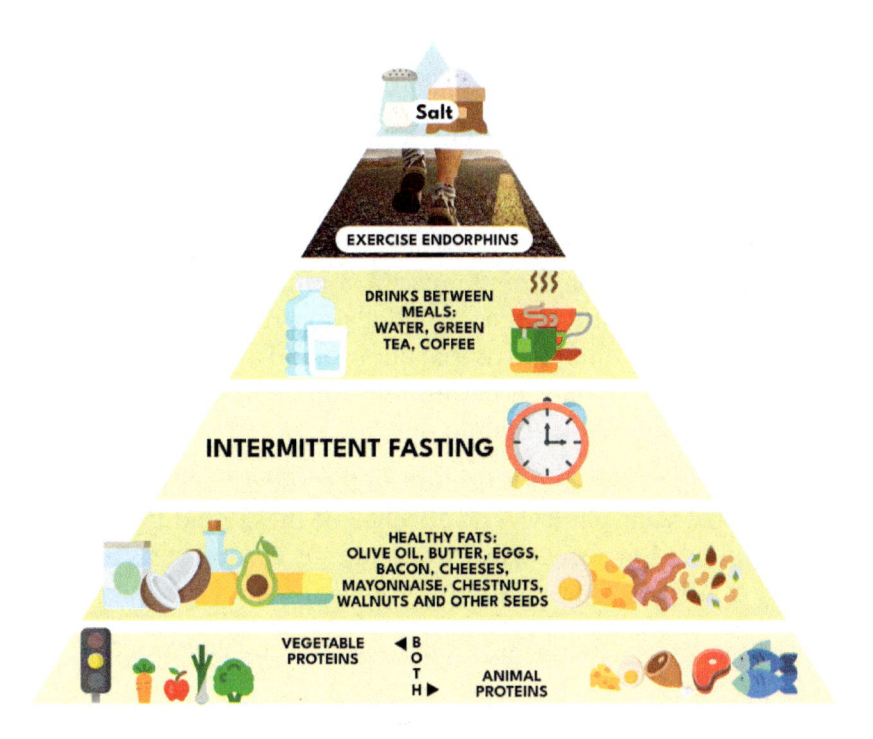

Table 1 - Ketogenic pyramid

How do you start the ketogenic diet in practice?

Choice of food:

The easiest way is to clean your kitchen of non-ketogenic foods that contain carbohydrates. You should think of protein first and healthy fat as energy. After all, as already explained, you can extract energy from both carbohydrates and fat. However, since we only use fat when there are no carbohydrates, we must eliminate carbohydrates from our diet. Successful dietary re-education requires a change in mentality, forgetting other nutritional advice, and avoiding food fads. You don't have to be afraid of eating fat; don't mix dietary concepts from other diets with the ketogenic diet.

Choosing the right food is not limited to the supermarket. You also need to organize your pantry. The absence of these readily available foods at home will prevent you from slipping up unnecessarily. So we will say goodbye to the following foods.

- To the garbage with the flours and starch (wheat, corn, and cassava).
- Bye-bye to sugary drinks like soda and fruit juice.
- Goodbye to sugar, honey, and fruits.
- Say *adios* to ice cream, sweets, and cakes.
- Do not eat fruit except small portions of strawberries.
- Say *arrivederci* to grains and legumes (beans, lentils, chickpeas, peas, potatoes, corn, rice).
- Don't use oils with omega 6 (sunflower, corn, wheat), as excess intake contributes to inflammation and oxidative stress[106].
- Do not drink alcohol, as it contains carbohydrates and stores energy. Many alcoholic drinks can knock you out of ketosis.
- In general, it is recommended to avoid industrial trans fatty acids. Avoid margarine and processed vegetable oils.

Go to the supermarket yourself (don't delegate, as awareness is essential, and with knowledge of the food, it's more likely to work) and buy ketogenic foods, constantly checking the nutritional information. Next, we will teach you how to read the nutritional table correctly and make your own decisions.

- Use olive oil, chestnuts, walnuts (in moderation), *psyllium*, whole eggs (prefer organic), mushrooms, coconut oil, lard, and apple cider vinegar.
- Milk and butter have conjugated linoleic acid, which has been shown to increase HDL and potentially reduce inflammation[xxviii].
- Beef, poultry, pork, chicken, turkey, duck, sausage, salami, ham, hamburger and bacon.
- Fish and seafood:
    - Tuna, sardines, and salmon, which are rich in omega-3.
    - Trout.
    - Tilapia.
    - Shrimp.
    - Scallops.
    - Lobster.
- Leafy greens, 2 cups per day (measured raw):
    - Lettuce.
    - Cress.
    - Chard.
    - Cabbage.
    - Spinach.
    - Arugula.
    - Cabbage.
- Fruit:
    - Avocado.
    - Strawberry and red fruits in small quantities.
- Non-starchy vegetables, 1 cup per day (measured raw):

[xxviii] Dietary inflammation depends on many other factors, which I discuss in my book Strategic Anti-inflammatory Diet (https://bio.amato.io/dieta)

- Amaranth or Chinese spinach.
- Artichoke.
- Artichoke hearts.
- Asparagus.
- Corn.
- Bamboo shoots.
- Beans.
- Bean sprouts.
- Beet leaves.
- Brussels sprouts.
- Broccoli.
- Cabbage.
- Carrots.
- Cauliflower.
- Celery.
- Cucumber.
- Eggplant.
- Cabbage.
- Mustard.
- Turnip.
- Leek.
- Mushrooms.
- Okra.
- Onions.
- Pod.
- Pepper.
- Radish.
- Green salad (chicory, endive, lettuce, spinach, arugula, radish, watercress).
- Peas.
- Chard.
- Tomato.

• Foods that are permitted on a limited basis[xxix]

[xxix] Portions should not be added together, but rather considered as alternatives.

- Cheese: up to 120ml. It includes hard, aged, cheddar, brie, camembert, mozzarella, gruyere, cream cheese and goat cheese. But pay attention to the amount of carbohydrates that some may contain.
  - Creams, oils, and butter: 2 tablespoons per day.
  - Mayonnaise: 2 tablespoons per day.
  - Olives: up to 6 per day.
  - Avocado: half a fruit per day.
  - Lemon/Lime: 2 tablespoons per day.
  - Soy sauce: 2 tablespoons per day.
  - Pickles: 2 per day.
- Pasta:
  - Konjac[xxx]
  - Peach palm
- Snacks:
  - Zero-carb snacks (dehydrated parmesan cheese, cured meats, turkey breast) (no limit).
    - Avoid nuts as they can be eaten uncontrollably despite being low in carbohydrates.
  - Sugar-free gelatin.
  - Carpaccio.
  - Boiled eggs.
  - Pork rinds (from the microwave) can help initially, but you will soon realize that even if you like them, you will not be able to overeat them.
  - Sweeten, preferably with stevia.

[xxx] The Asian plant of the genus Amorphophallus konjac is widely used in Japanese cuisine. The root contains a non-digestible dietary fiber called glucomannan, also known as konjac mannan. When glucomannan is ingested, its fibers absorb water and thus increase in volume, giving a feeling of satiety. Some people report diarrhea.

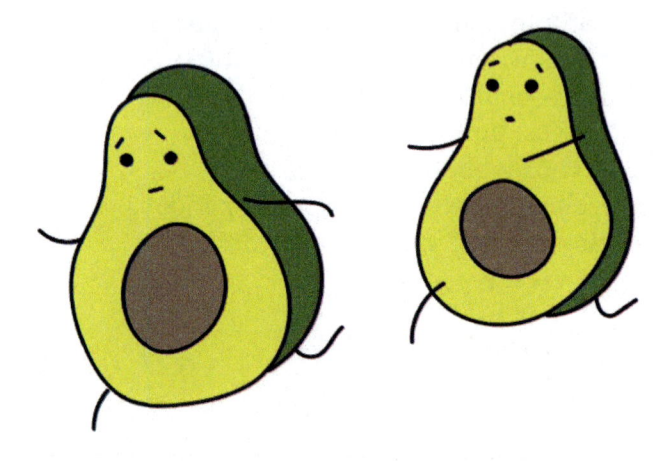

"I told you it's good fat!"

Do not avoid fat in real food. Reduce the amount of cream, oil, and fat to lose weight. By adding fat, you must burn that fat before you can start burning your own. Eat meals full of nutrients. See some examples:

Breakfast: Breakfast is unnecessary, but you can make an omelet, bacon, boiled eggs with cold-cut rolls, and coffee with healthy fats.

Lunch: there's nothing special about a ketogenic lunch. You'll eat meat, vegetables, or mushrooms sautéed in butter or coconut fat, olives, and salads with olive oil. It is an ordinary, tasty lunch without flour, grains, or legumes.

Dinner: you can repeat lunch or breakfast. Make cream, avocado, lemon, and coconut creams if you prefer something sweet. Later, you can take your chances with some ketogenic sweets.

In the initial phase, especially before entering ketosis, you may feel a desire for sweets.

Understand that a critical indicator of being in ketosis is a reduced craving for sweets. This change is biological and happens naturally over time.

When your body is no longer a sugar machine, it will naturally no longer need sugar.

You will discover that your addiction to sweets was nothing more than your body insatiably asking for energy.

As with the ketogenic diet, your body is powered by fat. So, in a month or two, you will start to crave cheese, salami, eggs, and butter. Your body will ask for fats, and you will gladly give them.

Unlike other dietary strategies, counting calories, proteins, and fats is unnecessary. However, it is essential to remove carbohydrates altogether. Do not exceed 20g of net carbs (or 50g of total carbs). Use the Taco table (https://bio.amato.io/taco) to plan your consumption, read the nutritional table of foods, or use an app dedicated to the ketogenic diet.

If you do not lose weight initially, reduce carbohydrates even further.

Over the weeks, you will learn how to measure your daily protein (eat enough to ensure nutrients and preserve lean mass), how to measure your fat intake (eat enough to keep losing weight), and your calories.

It is essential to say that you cannot eat excess calories due to the satiety induced by ketosis.

With two meals daily and ketogenic foods, exceeding the calorie count is challenging. As the desire to eat disappears in the first few weeks, you cannot do it even if you want to.

Avoid adding extra fat to your food when it's not needed. Specifically, this refers to avoiding 'fat bombs' – snacks that are primarily made of fat and often used in ketogenic diets. Additionally, Bulletproof coffee, which is coffee enriched with healthy fats, is not advantageous for a ketogenic diet despite being popularly recommended.

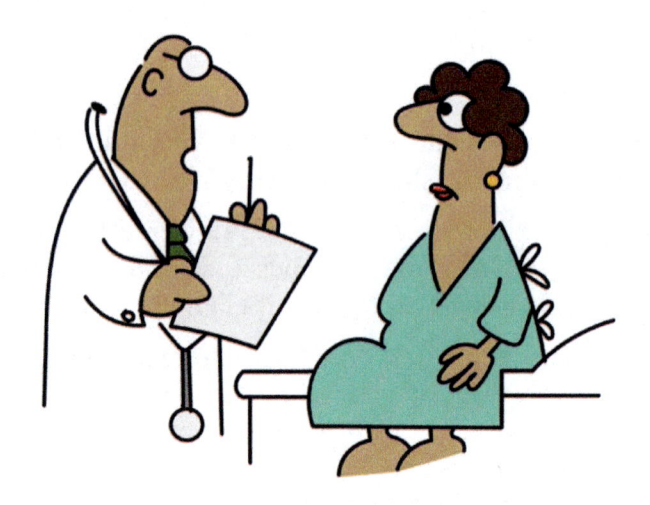

"The ketogenic diet is bad for you. I have a patient who slipped on some bacon and broke his leg."

How to prepare ketogenic meals quickly
One of the biggest self-sabotages is the excuse that you don't have the time or inclination to prepare your food. Don't give up when you don't have the inspiration to make a complete meal with several dishes. Make a quick meal by putting all the ingredients in a pan, frying pan, or bowl.

Cold meal	Leftovers	Hot meal	Meal with ground beef	Roast meal
Leftover cooked meat.	Leftover cooked meat.	Raw or cooked meat of any kind.	Defrosted raw ground beef.	Chicken thigh or wing, fish fillet, or pork loin.
Leftover raw or cooked vegetables or low-carb vegetables.	Fresh or frozen low-carb vegetables.	Fresh or frozen low-carb vegetables.	Fresh or frozen low-carb vegetables.	Vegetables that are well roasted: broccoli, cauliflower, carrots, radishes, or Italian zucchini.
Olive oil, nuts, or seeds.	Olive oil, coconut oil, or avocado.	Olive oil, coconut oil, avocado, or lard.	Olive oil, coconut oil, avocado, or lard.	Olive oil, coconut oil, avocado, or lard.
Vinegar, mayonnaise, lemon juice, or your favorite herbs and seasonings.	Favorite herbs and seasonings.	Bone broth or coconut milk (good for curries) + favorite herbs and seasonings.	Favorite herbs and seasonings, vinegar, or lemon juice.	Favorite herbs and seasonings.
Mix everything in a bowl, and it is ready.	Mix everything in a saucepan or frying pan, cover, and cook for around 10 minutes.	Mix everything in a saucepan or frying pan, cover, and heat until it boils. Then, reduce the temperature and leave for another 10 minutes or until thoroughly cooked.	Fry the ground meat in a saucepan or frying pan over medium heat until it turns pink. Add the vegetables and leave for another 10 minutes until completely cooked.	Preheat the oven to 205°C. Add vegetables to the fat and coat the meat with seasoning. Place everything in a suitable container and bake for 25 to 30 minutes until completely cooked.

What is the best cooking oil?

One of the biochemistry classes I remember most at medical school was the day I arrived late, and the laboratory smelled of "pastel de feira[xxxi]." It took me a while to understand that the teacher was

---

[xxxi] Brazilian market-style fried pastry, commonly known as "pastel de feira" in Brazil, is a popular street food item often found in local markets. It's a thin, crisp pastry made from a simple dough, filled with a variety of ingredients like seasoned ground beef, mozzarella cheese, heart of palm, or even shrimp, then deep-fried until golden and crispy. The outer crust is light and flaky, providing a delightful contrast to the savory, sometimes slightly spicy, filling inside. It's typically enjoyed

demonstrating the structural change in fat after heating it, and the smell of the pastry was the result of this change. Lard and olive oil are rich in monounsaturated fats and are, therefore, the best options for cooking, reducing the production of aldehydes. A tip for those using lard is to use fresh pancetta and make it at home instead of buying it in the supermarket. When we cook at high temperatures (>180°C), the molecular structures change, and oxidation occurs, which produces some toxic substances. Animal fats (lard and butter) and olive oil rarely oxidize. Avoid fried foods, especially at very high temperatures. If you are frying something, try to use as little oil as possible and try to remove any excess with a paper towel after frying. Olive oil has 76% monounsaturated, 14% saturated, and 10% polyunsaturated lipids, regardless of whether extra virgin. Olive oil, especially extra virgin olive oil, has proved to be very resistant to high temperatures and oxidation[107].

Is intermittent fasting necessary?

Use the intermittent fasting strategy intelligently. If you are accustomed to it, or if it's easy for you, then go ahead and take advantage of it. However, if you come from a life with lots of carbohydrate-filled snacks, you cannot start eating twice a day instantly. Do not worry. The satiety of ketosis comes with time, and you will naturally skip meals without realizing it. After this period, your body won't need to eat as much as before. Allow this to happen gradually and naturally.

How many meals should I eat a day?

Begin by eating three meals a day: breakfast, lunch, and dinner, without any snacks in between. Aim to have an early dinner and delay your breakfast as much as possible. This practice is your initial

---

as a quick snack or a casual meal, often accompanied by a cold beverage, and is a staple at Brazilian outdoor markets and food stalls.

step towards incorporating intermittent fasting. Don't push yourself too hard, even if rapid weight loss is your goal. It's not required. As previously mentioned, you will naturally start to feel more satiated.

If you continue to feel hungry throughout the day, increase the fats and proteins (be sensible) in your main meals.

If you're still hungry, try snacks like avocado, cheese, slices of bacon, quail eggs, and a few nuts. They can quickly get out of control. To minimize the risk, choose those without salt or, of course, sugar. They are less addictive. Do not be hungry. Never be hungry on the ketogenic diet. That's the great thing about the ketogenic diet: you can eat as much as you like, as long as you don't eat any carbohydrates.

How long does it take to get into ketosis?
The time varies greatly according to your dedication, history, and dependence on carbohydrates: your obesity, hormonal problems, metabolism, insulin, and your precision in withdrawing from carbohydrates. Remember that your body will need to adapt to produce ketone bodies efficiently. Often, this mechanism has been switched off for decades. But rest assured, it exists. When you are ready, you will enter ketosis. The average time is three to seven days.

What will I feel during the adaptation phase?
The most common adaptation symptoms are tiredness, cramps, sleepiness, tingling, headache, irritation, weakness, stomach pain, insomnia, muscle pain, and sugar cravings. The sensation can be similar to a cold. This adaptation phase can last from a few days to a month. But there is no need to feel this discomfort. You need to maximize your intake of foods with potassium, calcium, magnesium, and sodium (cheese, yogurt, sardines, almonds, walnuts). They will be missing from your diet initially. Hydration must be rigorous at the beginning as, many times, the symptoms simply arise from a lack of water for our metabolism to function correctly.

Once you have decided to start the diet, take it seriously to get the best results. Remember that escapes in the adaptation phase simply restart the process of entering ketosis, prolonging accommodation. With increased diuresis, your body will filter immense amounts of water, losing salts. Therefore, when you must replace minerals and electrolytes, increase your salt consumption. It is the only situation, and very temporary, in which I recommend increasing salt.

Have you started to feel any of the symptoms? Increase your salt and water consumption.

Sleep well by practicing sleep hygiene. Once you are ketogenic-adapted, you will notice an increase in energy, often waking up earlier naturally. But, in the initial adaptation phase, you must ensure seven to eight hours of sleep per day with good quality sleep.

Avoid or minimize external and internal stress. This means all possible stress on your body, whether it is a spike in blood sugar, a maddening routine, or grueling hours at the gym.

Eat enough protein. The ketogenic diet is not protein-restricted. It is a protein consumption adequacy diet. If you are experiencing symptoms, increase your consumption of fish, cheese, eggs, and meat.

Eat enough fats without adding fats unnecessarily. Ketogenic requires the consumption of good fats in high quantities. Sauté food in butter and coconut fat, and add olive oil to the salad. A small handful of chestnuts, walnuts, or macadamias daily can help.

If necessary, supplement vitamins and minerals. Try to consume the foods that will do this for you. If it is not enough, see your doctor.

How do I know if I'm in ketosis?

Once you have gone through the adaptation period, you will start to feel the classic symptoms: dry mouth, bad breath (the keto habit is temporary), more energy, and almost non-existent hunger are all indicative of ketosis.

The most accurate way to make sure you are in ketosis is to use blood or breath-measuring devices. Use it when you start to feel the symptoms I mentioned above.

- Mild nutritional ketosis (weight loss): between 0.5 mmol/L and 1.0 mmol/L.
- Optimal ketosis (cognitive benefits and physical performance): between 1.0 mmol/L and 3.0 mmol/L.
- Therapeutic ketosis: between 3.0 mmol/L and 6.0 mmol/L.

Measurements can also be taken in the laboratory, although the delay in response makes their use for practicing the ketogenic diet unfeasible.

Over time, you will naturally learn to diagnose physiological ketosis by observing changes in your body.

However, this is not a guarantee that you are in ketosis or that your ketone bodies have reached an ideal number for you.

How long should I follow the ketogenic diet?

There is no scientific evidence of long-term harm from the ketogenic diet.

Even if you read about supposed fatigue or nutritional deficiencies on the ketogenic diet, note that these studies are questionable. It all depends on the food variety introduced into your diet. Nutritional deficiency can occur when trying to combine calorie restriction with maintaining ketogenic status, which can result in a poorly balanced diet with nutritional deficiency. Never try to incorporate a ketogenic diet with a low-calorie diet without professional supervision.

The problem is not the ketogenic diet. The solution is not to get off it, but to improve your diet. Therefore, a lot of quality is required in the selected foods.

We recommend that your doctor and nutritionist monitor the long-term diet.

Sustainability of the ketogenic diet

Carbophilia is an addiction to carbohydrates, and obesity is a direct effect of this lifestyle. Carbohydrates are highly addictive, like neuroactive drugs that create instant euphoria and tranquility followed by feelings of negativity, guilt, harm, and repression. Just remember children that when they eat sugar, they get agitated.

Obesity in carbohydrate addicts should be viewed like alcoholism in Alcoholics Anonymous. The unhealthy relationship with carbohydrates must be recognized, and the goal must be total abstinence from them.

It is necessary to understand that it is not a punitive, restrictive, or temporary diet. You deserve better, and the best is not carbohydrates. You can enjoy a menu of authentic, healthy foods from the land and ocean.

Have a dietary plan for foods you can produce, purchase from supermarkets or restaurants, or eat with friends and family while traveling and on vacation. Always have "emergency" ketogenic foods for times of need, such as snacks or quick meals, so you don't use momentary tiredness as an excuse to slip up.

The perfect is the enemy of the done. Do not seek perfection but relatively constant progress. When you make a mistake, don't blame yourself. Learn from your mistakes.

Take responsibility, analyze your mistakes, and correct them. You may stumble but return to your previous position. Have resilience; don't let life's fluctuations affect your decision. Be tolerant of frustrations; don't dwell on them.

Be proud of your efforts, and celebrate your victories. Think and meditate on your emotions so they don't interfere with your conscious decisions.

Practice healthy habits and replace your old unhealthy habits. It doesn't have to be everything simultaneously, but you must remember a replacement sequence.

Be good enough and express gratitude and kindness to yourself and others throughout the day. Love yourself. Participating in a group to exchange experiences and support can help with the process in the long term.

How do you correctly read the nutritional table of foods?

Making healthy choices means much more than putting a product in the supermarket trolley that claims to be low-carb or ketogenic. Often, a product like this can be industrialized and over-processed to the point of being unhealthy. Instead, it is vital to know how to read the nutritional labels[xxxii] of foods and understand what all those numbers and information mean. It serves to inform the consumer about the composition of the food and the number of nutrients it provides, as well as indicating how much this represents of the recommended daily intake (% DV) for a healthy adult person who is not on any diet and follows the guidance published in law[xxxiii]. The nutritional information is typically found on the back of food packaging, often in small print and presented in a standardized, understated format. However, the inconspicuous presentation of this information does not reflect its significance. It is in these details that you can determine whether a food is healthy or not. This section is immune to marketing tactics, offering a straightforward representation of the product's contents.

The first piece of information you need to pay attention to interpret the nutritional table correctly is the serving size indicated by the manufacturer – which is usually only part of the total contents of the package, as the rest of the information will be proportional to that serving, and not to the entire food package. That's the first catch.

[xxxii] The nutritional table for food was regulated by Anvisa resolution 360/2003.
[xxxiii] RDC RESOLUTIONS NO. 269, OF SEPTEMBER 22, 2005 AND NO. 360, OF DECEMBER 23, 2003. Based on American publications that suggest the recommended daily intake of 75g protein, 55g total fat and 300g carbohydrates for adults.

For example, you might get excited thinking that a bar of chocolate has only 120 calories, as specified in the nutritional table, without realizing that this figure corresponds to only 20 grams (just four squares). So, if you consume the entire bar, usually 140 grams, you will ingest 840 calories! Here, you can calculate the total amount by using the rule of three[xxxiv].

Therefore, you should always look at the serving size in grams or milliliters to find out how much you can or should eat of each food and to be able to compare the nutritional value of various products.

The second trick is in the daily value (% DV), which shows the amount of the nutrient in question (carbohydrates, proteins, sodium, etc.) present in a serving of the product compared to the amount an average person should consume in a day on a standard, non-ketogenic diet. So bear in mind that this value changes according to individual needs. No one is an average person. Unique particularities must be considered. Remember that this is a reference based on the nutritional pyramid, which is constantly being questioned by the scientific community and does not reflect the proportion of macronutrients suggested in the ketogenic diet.

When considering a snack packet containing 120 kcal per 25 grams with a Daily Value (DV) of 6%, each serving size (approximately one and a half cups) contributes 6% of the recommended daily calorie intake for a diet of 2,000 calories.

However, if you're on a low-calorie diet and only consume 1,200 calories daily, that same serving represents 10% of your daily value.

In the nutritional table, carbohydrates appear in their own line. For those on the ketogenic diet, you should disregard the % DV information, as the aim is to remove carbohydrates from the meal and

---

[xxxiv] In mathematics, the rule of three is a way of finding a quantity that has the same relationship to another known quantity as it does to two other known numerical values. Two quantities are directly proportional when one increases in the same proportion as the other. In the example mentioned, it would be: $\frac{120}{20} = \frac{x}{140}$ multiplied by a cross would be $x = \frac{120 \times 140}{20} = \frac{16.800}{20} = 840$

only pay attention to the number of grams of carbohydrates per serving mentioned.

Take the example of a cracker that contains in the nutritional table (Table 3) the information of a 9g serving (1 packet) containing 6.1g of carbohydrates with a % DV of 2 (for someone on a 300g carbohydrate diet), for someone on a ketogenic diet of 20g/day of carbohydrates the % DV would be 32. Therefore, the % DV is not calculated for the ketogenic diet.

Table 3 - Nutritional table of crackers

NUTRITIONAL INFORMATION 9g serving (1 package)		
	Amount per serving	%DV(*)
Energetic Value	39kcal or 164kJ	2%
Carbohydrates	6.1g	2%
Proteins	1.1g	1%
Total fat	1.1g	2%
Saturated Fat	0.6g	3%
Trans Fats	0	**
Dietary Fiber	0	0%
Sodium	25 mg	1%
* % Daily Reference Values based on a 2000 kcal or 8400 kJ diet. Your daily values may be higher or lower depending on your energy needs. ** DV not established.		

Likewise, this will be the case with other nutrients. So, suppose you have any restrictions on your intake of sodium, sugars, fats, or, in the case of the ketogenic diet, carbohydrates. In that case, you need to consider your individual needs rather than the percentage of the standard daily value shown in the nutritional tables. These are suitable for people without any specific conditions. In our recipes below, we've included the nutritional table according to the recommended standards so that you can start practicing.

Energetic value
Concerning energy value, this is usually the first item in the table and means the amount of calories present in the serving. This value is

represented in kilocalories (kcal) and kilojoules (kJ). Kilocalories (kcal), popularly referred to as "calories," are the value we take into account in our daily lives, and this is what you should base yourself on. As 1 kcal equals 4184 kJ, this figure will always be much higher.

For the ketogenic diet, the energy value is not as significant as for those on a low-calorie diet because calorie restriction is not the aim of the ketogenic diet but rather metabolic change.

But it's interesting to understand that proteins, carbohydrates, and fats have different energy values (Table 4). You'll notice that the energy value of fats is higher than that of carbohydrates, making them an effective energy source for storage in our bodies. And it can help to break the myth that without carbohydrates, we have no energy for the body: in reality, fat is a source of energy.

Table 4 - Energetic value of macronutrients

	Energetic value
Carbohydrates	4 kcal/g - 17 kJ/g
fats	9 kcal/g - 37 kJ/g
Proteins	4 kcal/g - 17 kJ/g
Alcohol	7 kcal/g - 29 kJ/g

One food can be higher in calories and at the same time offer more nutrients and fiber, while another product can be lower in calories but low in nutrients and high in sodium – which is harmful for hypertensive people. Our bodies may poorly absorb other foods and, despite their properties, go unused, such as konjac potatoes[xxxv]. That's why it's essential to evaluate the whole package.

[xxxv] Konjac is grown in East Asia because it is a great source of starch and is used to create a flour and a paste of the same name. Its nutritional content is practically zero, but it does contain minerals. Its fibers are not digested by the body and pass straight through the digestive tract. Since it is low in calories, it is considered dietary, but since it is low in nutrients, you should avoid eating too much of it.

Carbohydrates

It is the sum of the sugars in food and is the primary macronutrient to avoid in the ketogenic diet. Carbohydrates that are not used for energy are stored as fat.

The primary carbohydrate sources are pasta, grains, breads, cereals, rice, corn, tubers, and sweets.

The ketogenic diet generally consists of **keeping carbohydrates below 20 grams** (about 0.7 ounces) daily. For comparison purposes, the very low carbohydrate diet is below 50 grams (about 1.76 ounces) a day, and the low carbohydrate diet (low carb) is below 100 grams (about 3.5 ounces) a day.

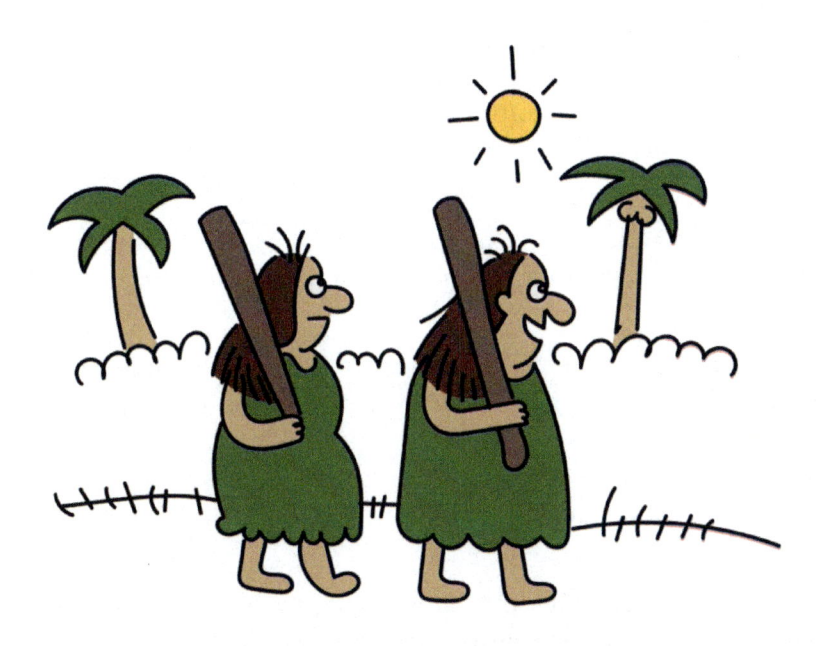

"Hunting and gathering doesn't seem profitable. Let's invent carbohydrates."

Proteins

These are the nutrients needed to build new tissues, such as muscles, and to regenerate cells and organs. Proteins are found mainly in foods of animal origin, such as meat, eggs, milk, and dairy products, but they are also present in legumes.

Proteins take longer to digest than carbohydrates. That's why they make you feel fuller. The daily protein requirement is generally 75 grams (0.8 to 1.5g per kilogram of body weight). Still, people who want to increase their muscle mass may have different needs (1.7 to 2.2g of protein per kilogram of body weight for healthy young people).[108–114]

If you're eating too little protein, you could lose muscle mass; if you're overdoing it, you could start gaining extra sugar.

In the ketogenic diet, there is no need to change the amount of protein in the usual diet, and therefore, the % DV can be within the values indicated on the labels.

Total fat

It is the sum of all the types of fat present in the serving of food, including polyunsaturated, monounsaturated, saturated, and trans fats.

Fats are necessary for the production and functioning of some hormones, for the metabolism of oily vitamins (A, D, E, and K), and for the support of tissues, and are the primary energy source in the ketogenic diet. For those seeking to lose weight, adding fats to the diet will increase the energy availability of the diet, delaying the use of body stores.

On the ketogenic diet, it's OK to eat a little extra fat. For example, coconut oil is rich in medium-chain triglycerides quickly converted into ketones.

The % DV of fats that appears in the nutritional table of foods is not comparable to that of those on the ketogenic diet.

Saturated fat

Saturated fats are found in foods of animal origin, such as meat, sausages, and whole dairy products. The ketogenic diet is naturally high in saturated fats. The subject here can be extensive and profound, involving many old and incomplete concepts and perpetuated myths being questioned and combated. Fats alone can be present in the disease and can be related to other harmful lifestyle habits, but this does not mean that they are the sole cause of the disease. Our hormones and many physiological processes essential for survival need fats to function correctly.

Trans fats

The most significant source of this type of fat is industrialized and highly processed foods with additional hydrogenated vegetable fat in their manufacture, such as margarine, packet snacks, microwave popcorn, chocolates, ice cream, and filled cookies.

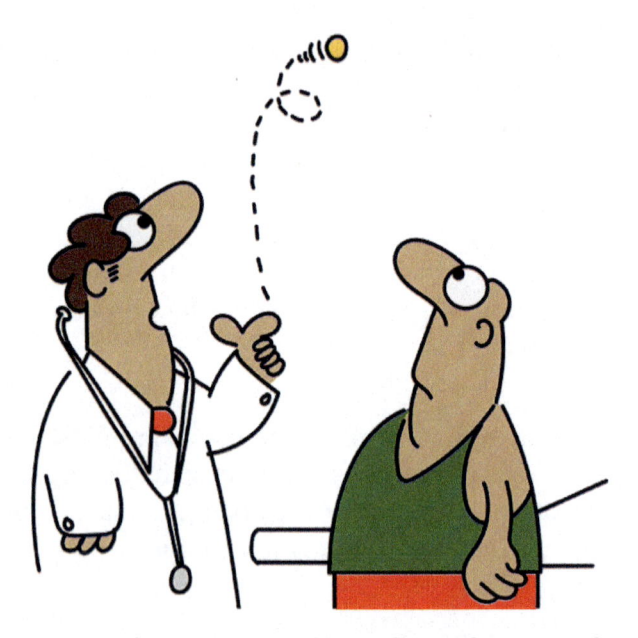

"Heads: fat is good and carbs are bad
Tails: fat is bad and carbohydrates
are good "

Dietary fiber

Fibers are non-digestible components found mainly in fruits, vegetables, and legumes and are essential for the proper functioning of the intestine. They contribute to increased fecal volume and intestinal motility and stimulate the development of beneficial bacteria that improve digestion and metabolism.

In addition, fiber reduces the speed at which carbohydrates are absorbed, promoting a glycemic control effect (amount of glucose in the blood) and reducing cholesterol absorption, helping to maintain healthy HDL and LDL levels.

By requiring more effort from the digestive system and forming a gel that expands in the stomach, fiber also prolongs the feeling of satiety, contributing to weight loss. The daily requirement is 25 grams.

By removing carbohydrate-rich foods from our diet, we often remove our daily sources of dietary fiber, which can cause constipation. We need dietary fiber such as arugula, spinach, eggplant, mushrooms, broccoli, cauliflower, zucchini, peppers, fennel, cabbage, asparagus, radish, lettuce, celery and kale. These low-carb vegetables are rich in fiber, vitamins, minerals, antioxidants, and much more. Starchy vegetables such as carrots, yams, beets, turnips, and sweet potatoes should be avoided.

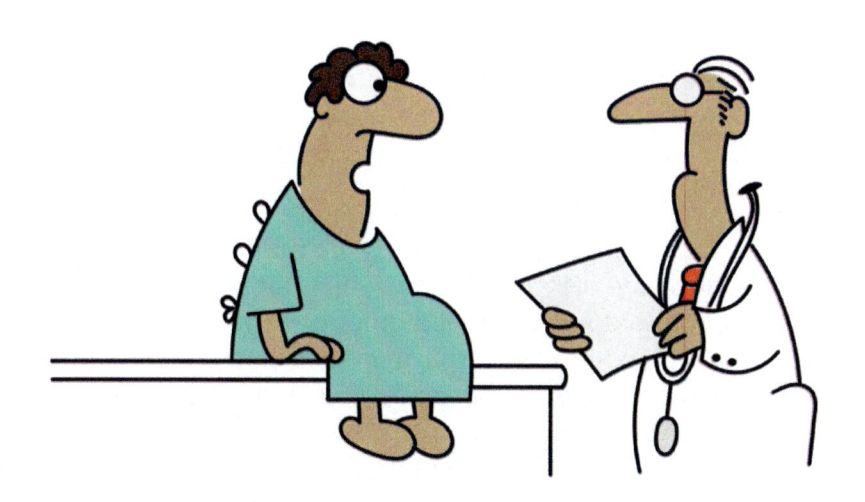

"Don't tell me to improve my diet. I ate a carrot once and nothing happened."

Sodium
It is a necessary mineral for performing various cellular functions, but its consumption should be restricted as it is directly related to increased blood pressure and kidney overload.

Although there are concerns about consuming table salt, an excellent sodium source, this mineral is also present in most processed foods, as it is a flavoring and preservation agent for these products.

The problem is that this sodium, which is often consumed without the person realizing it (in diet or zero sugar products, for example), can cause health damage. For this reason, we should also pay attention to the amount of this element shown in the nutritional table and avoid consuming more than the 2,400 mg recommended daily.

It's worth remembering that, as with other nutrients, the safe limit of sodium intake varies from person to person, so your needs and restrictions may differ. Sodium is recognized as a critical isolated cardiovascular risk factor and is being studied as an essential risk factor in women with lipedema[115,116].

Ingredient list
The list of ingredients, often placed above the nutritional table, is another excellent way of assessing food composition. The ingredients must be listed in descending order of their proportion in the food formulation. When a specific ingredient is prepared with two or more elements, it must be accompanied by a list in brackets and in descending order of proportion. It, therefore, serves not only to see what the formula contains but, above all, to identify the proportions between them. An example of the importance of the list comes from some "whole grain breads" that have more refined flour than whole grain in their composition, and also foods with many unrecognized chemicals in their composition. Additives to simulate food consistency in products that vaguely resemble natural food are very common.

The list makes it easy to identify foods you may be intolerant to (see Strategic Anti-inflammatory Diet) or even allergic to. But a beneficial rule of thumb is to look for lists that contain recognized foods and little or no unrecognized chemicals.

Conclusion:

There are countless fad diets, but few really take advantage of the way the human metabolism works. This is why the ketogenic diet persists, changing context and narrative but preserving the metabolic rationale. After all, it's easier or more exciting for humans to remember a captivating story than a list of permitted and forbidden foods. This book doesn't aim to bring you the latest fad diet but rather to present a well-established concept in an understandable scientific way, dispelling myths and fears that could prevent you from taking advantage of this benefit.

You may believe that a diet that allows (allows is different from encouraging) you to eat bacon[xxxvi], and your favorite cheeses can't work. Still, as soon as you flip the metabolic switch and turn your body into a machine that turns fat into energy naturally and efficiently with only natural resources, you realize that cheese is just one of the delicious possibilities. In the ketogenic diet, you don't need to count calories or weigh food, but you do need to understand its metabolic principle and know the composition of the food. Ketosis, although uncommon today, is a perfectly natural and healthy state of our bodies. Many of today's diseases can be caused by the absence of this state due to the inexhaustible supply of tasty foods with a high glycemic index.

Many people believe that carbohydrates are necessary for an energetic life. Still, science shows that the ketogenic diet is effective in losing fat and weight and bringing other benefits. By putting your body into ketosis, it will 'burn' fat for energy and prevent and treat diabetes, heart disease, lipedema, epilepsy, and other illnesses. Drink plenty of water to make the transition easier and avoid the

---

[xxxvi] Fried bacon is rich in nitrites and Advanced Glycation End Products (AGEs), both of which are linked to the development of cancer. Microwave-cooked bacon has lower levels of heterocyclic amines.

carbohydrates that tempt you. With some planning and preparation, you can have a smooth transition and benefit in the long run.

Here are several tasty and varied recipes with very low carbohydrates. These are suggestions that can be part of your ketogenic diet. Pay attention to the amount of carbohydrates in each and learn to use the nutritional information to your advantage. It will be a full plate for those who want a more practical approach.

Other books by the author

For all:

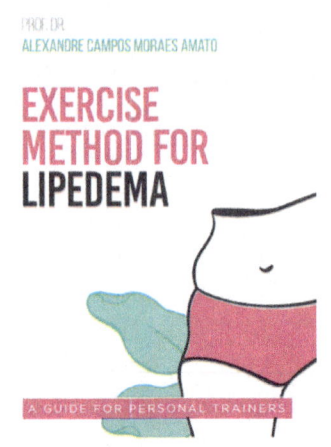

Discover relief from lipedema with "Exercise Method for Lipedema" by Dr. Alexandre Amato. This guide is crucial for individuals and educators seeking effective lipedema management strategies. Dr. Amato, a respected expert, offers a new exercise approach grounded in extensive research. Simple and adaptable, the book is a valuable tool for understanding and tackling lipedema. Get your copy today and embark on a journey towards improved health and well-being in the context of lipedema. https://bio.amato.io/method

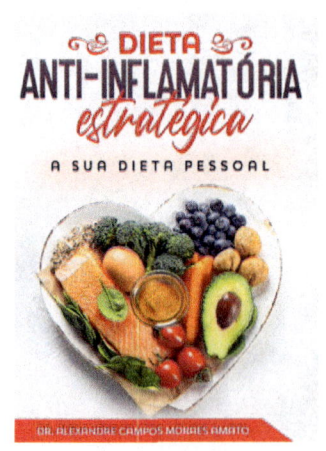

Strategic Anti-inflammatory Diet: your personal diet. Complete your nutritional knowledge with this book. Are you tired of looking for the ideal diet? Have you ever thought that there is no perfect diet that fits everyone? When you think about healthy eating, do you know what healthy means? What if your idea of "healthy" was ingrained in you by someone who wants to sell a product? If it is healthy for you, is it healthy for everyone? But if no off-the-shelf diet works for everyone, how do you find out which foods are the healthiest for you? Stop being driven to fad diets, which may work for some people but not necessarily for you. Learn how to judge which foods are healthy. Understand how to drastically improve your quality of life by treating your symptoms. Understand how to go through the self-knowledge phase and have a real and customized strategy to impact your life positively. Re-educate yourself! https://bio.amato.io/dieta

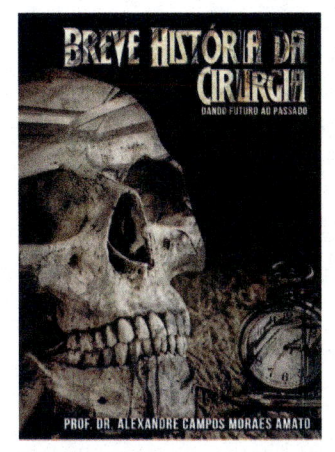

A Brief History of Surgery: This book recalls, in an abridged form, the most critical moments that led to the current development of surgery in Brazil and the world. Important surgeons, exciting discoveries, trivia, and the pillars of modern surgery. The History of Medicine focuses on invasive procedures, told concisely, objectively, light, and fun. https://bio.amato.io/historia-cirurgia

For healthcare professionals:

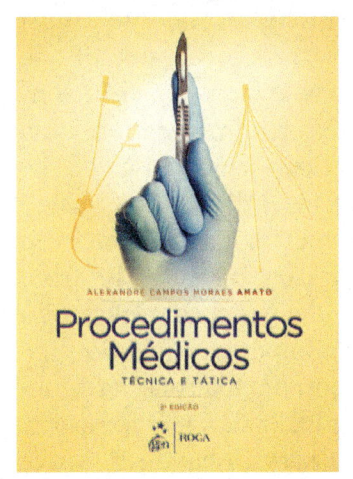

Medical Procedures - Technique and Tactics. Even the simplest medical procedures can risk a patient's life, so they must be conducted cautiously and precisely. These are the aspects that guided the conception of this work. Medical Procedures | Technique and Tactics, fully revised and improved in its second edition, presents the best technologies for each clinical situation, from patient preparation and care to possible errors that put patients at risk. Its 83 chapters are divided into 14 sections and standardized by topics, covering the main items for performing each procedure. They include illustrations of the materials and step-by-step techniques. This book is both theoretical and practical, suitable for students, nurses, surgeons, and other healthcare professionals. https://bio.amato.io/procedimentos

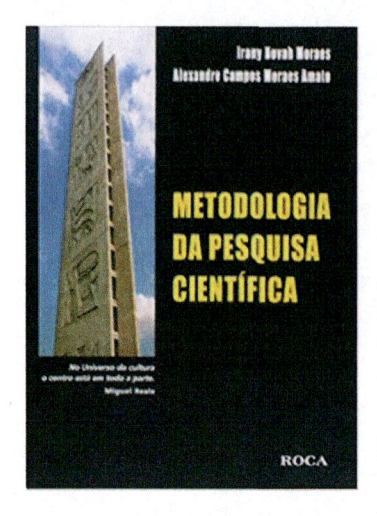

Scientific Research Methodology. Scientific investigation, or scientific research, has its norms and rules, which are the paths that lead to the study's success. This publication aims to clearly and simply show these avenues in the field of science, helping with all the stages of scientific research methodology: planning, preparation, completion, right through to the final presentation.

https://bio.amato.io/metodologia

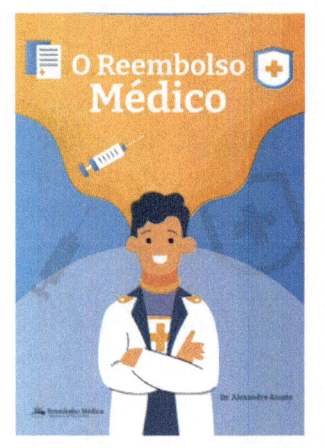

Medical Reimbursement is the most innovative way to work professionally in healthcare. The balance between decision-making power, medical information, and financial power allows medicine to be carried out without the influence of vested interests. It is suitable for the patient, who receives health information directly from the source, without the economic filter of a health insurance company, and for the doctor, whose recommendations are not influenced by a health insurance company. And for this relationship to work, it is necessary to have resolutive and high-quality medical care, requirements that are beneficial to the health insurance company. Medical Reimbursement is healthy for everyone involved, so this book teaches how to apply it in daily practice. It makes it possible to understand how the healthcare service model and its financing works. Without this knowledge, the doctor becomes dependent on intermediaries, who specialize in diminishing the importance and value of the doctor himself. Every medical professional should know how Medical Reimbursement

works, their rights, and patients' rights to help them in every way.
https://bio.amato.io/livro-reembolso

Ketogenic recipes

Breakfast
Creamy Chicken Pancake

NUTRITIONAL INFORMATION		
30g serving (1/4 of the unit)		
	Amount per serving	%DV(*)
Energetic value	70kcal or 297kJ	3%
Carbohydrates	1.6g	1%
Proteins	5.7g	8%
Total fat	4.5g	8%
Saturated fat	1.7g	8%
Trans fats	0g	**
Dietary fiber	0.8g	3%
Sodium	107 mg	4%

* % Daily Reference Values based on a 2000 kcal or 8400 kJ diet. Your daily values may be higher or lower depending on your energy needs.
** DV not established.

Yield: 1 serving

Preparation time: 20 minutes

Ingredients

- 1 egg white
- 1 egg
- 1 dessertspoonful of chia seeds
- 1 tablespoon of almond flour
- 2 tablespoons of grated parmesan cheese
- 1 pinch of turmeric
- Fine herbs
- 1 tablespoon of cream
- 80g chicken breast pre-seasoned with garlic, lemon and salt

Preparation method

Cook the chicken with some water and saffron; let the meat cool and shred it.

Add chicken, cream, and fine herbs.

Mix the egg, cheese, chia, and flour in a container.

Add the pancake mix and brown both sides in a non-stick frying pan.

Fill the pancake with the chicken and fold it over.

Tuna Protein Cake
Yield: 6 servings
Preparation time: 30 minutes

Ingredients

- 1 can of diet tuna
- 1 egg
- 2 tablespoons of flaxseed flour
- 2 tablespoons of natural yogurt
- ½ lemon squeezed
- Parsley to taste
- Black pepper to taste
- Coconut oil and flour for greasing

Preparation method
Mix all the ingredients.
Place in cupcake tins greased with coconut oil and flour, or, if the consistency allows, make balls and place on a (greased) baking sheet, bake for 20 minutes. You can also put it in the air fryer.

NUTRITIONAL INFORMATION 60g serving (1 unit)			
	Amount per serving	%DV(*)
Energetic value	118kcal or 495kJ	6
Carbohydrates	5.2g	2
Proteins	12g	16
Total fat	5.5g	10
Saturated fat	1.2g	5
Trans fats	-	**
Dietary fiber	1g	4
Sodium	139 mg	6

* % Daily Reference Values based on a 2000 kcal or 8400 kJ diet. Your daily values may be higher or lower depending on your energy needs.
** DV not established.

Guacamole
Yield: 500g
Preparation time: 10 minutes

Ingredients

- ½ avocado or mashed avocado
- 2 tablespoons of olive oil
- 2 lemons squeezed
- 2 crushed garlic cloves
- Salt and black pepper to taste

Preparation method

Mix all the ingredients well until they become a paste. If necessary, add a few more ingredients until it tastes just right. If stored in the refrigerator, it lasts for 3 to 4 days.

NUTRITIONAL INFORMATION		
60g serving (3 tablespoons)		
	Amount per serving	%DV(*)
Energetic value	60kcal or 250kJ	3
Carbohydrates	2.1g	1
Proteins	0.4g	-
Total fat	5.5g	10
Saturated fat	0.9g	4
Trans fats	-	**
Dietary fiber	1.5g	6
Sodium	-	-

* % Daily Reference Values based on a 2000 kcal or 8400 kJ diet. Your daily values may be higher or lower depending on your energy needs.
** DV not established.

Turkey Breast Basket
Yield: 6 servings
Preparation time: 15 minutes

Ingredients

- 6 slices of turkey breast
- 6 whole eggs
- Parsley and salt to taste
- Coconut oil (for greasing)

Preparation method

Grease cupcake tins with coconut oil, place a slice of turkey breast in each tin, break an egg on top of each slice, and sprinkle the seasoning. Place in the oven, turn off as soon as the egg is cooked (to your taste).

NUTRITIONAL INFORMATION			
74g serving (1 unit)			
	Amount per serving	%DV(*)
Energetic value	125kcal or 525kJ	6
Carbohydrates	1.4g	-
Proteins	14g	19
Total fat	6.8g	12
Saturated fat	1.9g	9
Trans fats	-	**
Dietary fiber	0.6g	2
Sodium	300 mg	12

* % Daily Reference Values based on a 2000 kcal or 8400 kJ diet. Your daily values may be higher or lower depending on your energy needs.
** DV not established.

Eggs with Mushrooms
Yield: 2 servings
Preparation time: 20 minutes

Ingredients

- 2 tablespoons of butter
- 250 g mushrooms, sliced
- 4 eggs
- Salt and black pepper to taste

Preparation method

In a saucepan or frying pan, melt 1 tablespoon of butter and cook the mushrooms until they are soft and darker. Set aside. In a non-stick frying pan, melt the other tablespoon of butter and add the beaten eggs. Stir with a spoon and cook until firm but still soft. Serve the eggs and mushrooms while still warm.

NUTRITIONAL INFORMATION			
245g serving (1 unit)			
	Amount per serving		%DV(*)
Energetic value	360kcal or 1,512kJ		18
Carbohydrates	7.6g		2
Proteins	15g		20
Total fat	30g		54
Saturated fat	14g		64
Trans fats	-		**
Dietary fiber	3g		12
Sodium	772 mg		32
* % Daily Reference Values based on a 2000 kcal or 8400 kJ diet. Your daily values may be higher or lower depending on your energy needs. ** DV not established.			

Chicken Soufflé
Preparation time: 30 minutes
Yield: 3 servings

Ingredients

- 100 g of shredded chicken
- 1 egg
- 1 egg white
- Parsley
- Basil
- 1 tablespoon of tomato cubes
- 1 tablespoon of cottage cheese
- Parmesan to finish (optional)

Preparation method
Preheat the oven to 200°C.
Beat the egg and white until they are uniform.
Place the chicken mixed with the spices and tomatoes in a baking dish.

Pour the egg mixture over the top.
Finish with cottage cheese and Parmesan.
Bake for 20 minutes or until golden brown.

NUTRITIONAL INFORMATION		
90g serving (1 unit)		
	Amount per serving	%DV(*)
Energetic value	122kcal or 512kJ	6
Carbohydrates	1g	-
Proteins	18g	24
Total fat	5.1g	9
Saturated fat	2.5g	11
Trans fats	-	**
Dietary fiber	-	-
Sodium	149 mg	6
* % Daily Reference Values based on a 2000 kcal or 8400 kJ diet. Your daily values may be higher or lower depending on your energy needs. ** DV not established.		

Scrambled Eggs with Leek and Parmesan
Yield: 2 servings
Preparation time: 10 minutes

Ingredients

- 2 whole eggs
- 1 tablespoon grated Parmesan
- 1 tablespoon of skimmed milk
- 1 cup of sliced leeks
- Salt and pepper to taste

Preparation method

Cut the leek into slices, the white part. Beat the eggs with the milk, add the leek, and season with salt and pepper. Heat a non-stick frying pan with a bit of olive oil or light butter and pour in the mixture. Let it cook, stirring constantly.

NUTRITIONAL INFORMATION			
110g serving (1 unit)			
	Amount per serving	%DV(*)
Energetic value	107kcal or 448kJ	5
Carbohydrates	3.9g	1
Proteins	8.6g	11
Total fat	6.3g	11
Saturated fat	2.4g	11
Trans fats	-	**
Dietary fiber	1.1g	4
Sodium	117 mg	5

* % Daily Reference Values based on a 2000 kcal or 8400 kJ diet. Your daily values may be higher or lower depending on your energy needs.
** DV not established.

Omelet of the Gods

Yield: 1 serving
Preparation time: 15 minutes

Ingredients

- 2 eggs
- 1 cup of grated semi-cured Minas cheese
- ¼ chopped onion
- ½ chopped tomato
- ½ cup of spinach
- Salt, black pepper, and olive oil to taste

Preparation method

Heat the oil in a frying pan, add the onion, tomato, spinach, and sauté—season with salt and pepper and set aside.

In a bowl, break the eggs and season with salt and pepper, stirring with a whisk or fork.

In the same frying pan where you prepared the vegetables, add more olive oil, heat it up, and add the eggs. Mix the contents of the pan a little with a fork so that it covers the pan's surface. When you notice that the underside is starting to brown and come away from the pan, turn off the heat, leaving your filling "creamy."

Add the sautéed vegetables and cheese to this creamy part, pulling the sides of the omelet together to form a small border so that the contents of the filling don't get lost. Turn the heat back on and slowly close the omelet.

To enjoy the creamy filling, serve immediately.

NUTRITIONAL INFORMATION			
145g serving (1/2 unit)			
	Amount per serving	%DV(*)
Energetic value	260kcal or 1,091kJ	13
Carbohydrates	5.2g	2
Proteins	17g	23
Total fat	19g	34
Saturated fat	10g	45
Trans fats	-	**
Dietary fiber	1.4g	6
Sodium	315 mg	13

* % Daily Reference Values based on a 2000 kcal or 8400 kJ diet. Your daily values may be higher or lower depending on your energy needs.
** DV not established.

Avocado Pate with Chicken

Yield: 5 servings
Preparation time: 5 minutes

Ingredients

- 2 tablespoons of avocado
- 1 lemon squeezed
- Mint leaves to taste
- ½ chopped tomato
- 1 tablespoon of shredded chicken

Preparation method

Clean the vegetables. Slice the tomatoes and mix with the avocado to form a smooth paste. Add the lemon and leave for 10 minutes to concentrate the flavor. Add the chicken and mix once more.

| NUTRITIONAL INFORMATION |||
| 60g serving (3 tablespoons) |||
	Amount per serving	%DV(*)
Energetic Value	58kcal or 245kJ	3
Carbohydrates	2.8g	1
Proteins	3.5g	5
Total fat	3.7g	7
Saturated fat	0.76g	3
Trans fats	-	**
Dietary fiber	2g	8
Sodium	3.7 mg	-

* % Daily Reference Values based on a 2000 kcal or 8400 kJ diet. Your daily values may be higher or lower depending on your energy needs.
** DV not established.

Ricotta and Chia Cheese Bread
Yield: 3 servings
Preparation time: 20 minutes

Ingredients

- 2 tablespoons of ricotta cream
- 1 cup of sour cassava starch
- ½ cup of ricotta
- 90 g of Greek-style yogurt
- 1 tablespoon of chia

Preparation method

Mix all the ingredients in a bowl until you have a very soft dough that doesn't stick to your hands (if necessary, add sprinkles to make it less sticky).

Form the balls and place them in the preheated oven at 180°C. Watch the dough rise and remove it when it becomes very brown.

NUTRITIONAL INFORMATION		
50g serving (1/2 unit)		
	Amount per serving	%DV(*)
Energetic value	180kcal or 756kJ	9
Carbohydrates	34g	11
Proteins	2.4g	3
Total fat	3.7g	7
Saturated fat	1.9g	9
Trans fats	-	**
Dietary fiber	0.6g	2
Sodium	136 mg	6
* % Daily Reference Values based on a 2000 kcal or 8400 kJ diet. Your daily values may be higher or lower depending on your energy needs. ** DV not established.		

Low Carb Pancake

Yield: 4 servings

Preparation time: 15 minutes

Ingredients

- 2 eggs
- 2 tablespoons of light cream cheese
- 1 tablespoon of grated parmesan cheese
- 1 pinch of salt
- 1 teaspoon of baking powder

Preparation method

Mix all ingredients in a blender. Pour the dough into a non-stick frying pan greased with olive oil and brown on both sides. Add the filling of your choice and cover with homemade tomato sauce.

| NUTRITIONAL INFORMATION |||
| 30g serving (1 unit) |||
	Amount per serving	%DV(*)
Energetic value	51kcal or 214kJ	3
Carbohydrates	0.71g	-
Proteins	4.2g	6
Total fat	3.5g	6
Saturated fat	1.7g	8
Trans fats	-	**
Dietary fiber	-	-
Sodium	236 mg	10

* % Daily Reference Values based on a 2000 kcal or 8400 kJ diet. Your daily values may be higher or lower depending on your energy needs.
** DV not established.

Low Carb Bread
Yield: 6 servings
Preparation time: 40 minutes

Ingredients

- 3 eggs
- 1 cup of almond flour
- 50 grams of grated parmesan cheese
- 3 tablespoons of water
- 3 tablespoons of cream
- 1 level tablespoon of baking powder

Preparation method

Place all the ingredients except the yeast in a blender and blend until smooth. Then, pour it into a bowl and mix in the yeast.

Pour the dough into a greased rectangular cake tin and bake at 200 degrees for 30 minutes or until golden brown.

Wait for it to cool down. Unmold and serve in slices.

NUTRITIONAL INFORMATION		
70g serving (1 unit)		
	Amount per serving	%DV(*)
Energetic value	197kcal or 827kJ	6
Carbohydrates	5.6g	2
Proteins	10g	13
Total fat	15g	27
Saturated fat	4.4g	20
Trans fats	-	**
Dietary fiber	2g	8
Sodium	541 mg	22
* % Daily Reference Values based on a 2000 kcal or 8400 kJ diet. Your daily values may be higher or lower depending on your energy needs. ** DV not established.		

Seed crisp

Yield: 30 servings
Preparation time: 30 minutes
Ingredients
- 1 cup of chia
- 1 cup of sunflower seeds (shelled and raw)
- 1 cup of white sesame
- 1 cup of Brazil nut flour
- 2 cups of water
- 1 pinch of salt to taste

Preparation method

Preheat the oven to 160 degrees and line the baking sheet with parchment paper. Mix all the ingredients, add the water, and stir well until the dough is thick. Wait a few minutes. Then, pour it into the pan and spread it until it becomes a thin layer. Make the cuts with a knife. Bake in a low oven for 30 minutes. Serve with garlic paste.

| NUTRITIONAL INFORMATION |||
| 30g serving (1 ½ unit) |||
	Amount per serving	%DV(*)
Energetic value	123kcal or 516kJ	6
Carbohydrates	4.9g	2
Proteins	3.8g	5
Total fat	9.8g	18
Saturated fat	1.5g	7
Trans fats	-	**
Dietary fiber	2.7g	11
Sodium	23 mg	1

* % Daily Reference Values based on a 2000 kcal or 8400 kJ diet. Your daily values may be higher or lower depending on your energy needs.
** DV not established.

Microwave Bread

Yield: 2 servings
Preparation time: 15 minutes

Ingredients

- 2 eggs
- 4 tablespoons of cream cheese
- 2 teaspoons of chemical yeast
- 1 dessert spoon of black (or white) sesame seeds
- Salt to taste
- Pepper to taste

Preparation method

Put all the ingredients except the sesame in a bowl and mix well until it forms a cream.

Spread in a large shallow dish (or divide into two small shallow dishes) and sprinkle with sesame seeds. Microwave for 1.5 minutes or until the "bread" is dry. Wait for it to cool down a little before handling. Suggestion: serve with hummus (chickpea paste) or cut into two pieces, fill to taste, and brown in the sandwich maker.

NUTRITIONAL INFORMATION			
95g serving (1 unit)			
	Amount per serving	%DV(*)
Energetic value	266kcal or 1,117kJ	13
Carbohydrates	4g	1
Proteins	13g	17
Total fat	22g	40
Saturated fat	12g	54
Trans fats	-	**
Dietary fiber	1.4g	6
Sodium	645 mg	27
* % Daily Reference Values based on a 2000 kcal or 8400 kJ diet. Your daily values may be higher or lower depending on your energy needs.			
** DV not established.			

Pancake with Chicken
Yield: 3 servings
Preparation time: 10 minutes

Ingredients

- 4 units of egg white
- 1 tablespoon of oat bran
- 1 pinch of salt and black pepper
- 5 tablespoons of cooked and shredded chicken (or sautéed ground beef)
- 2 tablespoons of tomato sauce
- 1 tablespoon of semi-cured cheese

Preparation method

Beat the egg whites with the oat bran, salt and pepper. Prepare the pancake in a medium non-stick frying pan greased with 1 drizzle of olive oil—Brown on both sides and stuff with shredded chicken (or ground beef). Serve with the sauce and grated cheese.

| NUTRITIONAL INFORMATION |||
| 145g serving (1 unit) |||
	Amount per serving	%DV(*)
Energetic value	133kcal or 559kJ	7
Carbohydrates	5.1g	2
Proteins	20g	27
Total fat	3.6g	7
Saturated fat	1.6g	7
Trans fats	-	**
Dietary fiber	1.1g	4
Sodium	283 mg	12

* % Daily Reference Values based on a 2000 kcal or 8400 kJ diet. Your daily values may be higher or lower depending on your energy needs.
** DV not established.

Yogurt Panna Cotta
Yield: 3 servings
Preparation time: 10 minutes

Ingredients

- 200 milliliters of coconut milk
- 1 teaspoon of agar-agar (or kanten)
- ½ cup of sweetener (xylitol)
- 400 milliliters of Greek yogurt
- ½ cup of organic strawberries
- ½ piece of lemon (just the juice)
- 1 dessert spoon of cinnamon powder
- ½ dessert spoon of powdered ginger
- Water (just enough to help beat)

Preparation method

Add the coconut milk, agar-agar, and xylitol in a pan and mix well. Bring to a boil, stirring constantly with a whisk (whisk) until it boils. After boiling, continue stirring continuously for another 3 minutes, turn off the heat, and wait for it to cool. Add the yogurt (which needs to be at room temperature), mixing constantly. Place the cream in glass jars and refrigerate for 30 minutes.

For the syrup:

Blend all the ingredients in a blender or food processor until you get a syrupy consistency. Pour the mixture over the pannacotta and refrigerate for 2 hours.

NUTRITIONAL INFORMATION 200g serving (1 unit)		
	Amount per serving	%DV(*)
Energetic value	390kcal or 1,599kJ	19
Carbohydrates	46g	15
Proteins	6.5g	9
Total fat	20g	36
Saturated fat	16g	73
Trans fats	-	**
Dietary fiber	2.9g	12
Sodium	85 mg	3

* % Daily Reference Values based on a 2000 kcal or 8400 kJ diet. Your daily values may be higher or lower depending on your energy needs.
** DV not established.

Protein Avocado
Yield: 3 servings
Preparation time: 5 minutes

Ingredients

- 1 small avocado
- ½ lemon
- 1 spoon of vanilla whey protein
- ½ glass of water
- 1 tablespoon of grated coconut for sprinkling

Preparation method

Mix all the ingredients in a blender until smooth—place in the refrigerator for at least an hour.

When serving, sprinkle the freshly grated coconut on top.

| NUTRITIONAL INFORMATION |||
| 60g serving (3 tablespoons) |||
	Amount per serving	%DV(*)
Energetic Value	81kcal or 340kJ	4
Carbohydrates	3.3g	1
Proteins	2.1g	3
Total fat	6.6g	12
Saturated Fat	1.8g	8
Trans fats	-	**
Dietary fiber	3g	12
Sodium	4.2 mg	-

* % Daily Reference Values based on a 2000 kcal or 8400 kJ diet. Your daily values may be higher or lower depending on your energy needs.
** DV not established.

Coconut Yogurt
Yield: 15 servings
Preparation time: 15 minutes

Ingredients

- 1 glass jar with lid
- 1 wooden spoon, tea towel, and elastic band
- 400 ml coconut milk
- 1 tablespoon of agar flakes or powder
- 1 probiotic capsule
- 1 teaspoon of vanilla extract (optional)
- 1 tablespoon of agave or syrup (optional)
- ½ lemon

Preparation method

Bring the coconut milk to the boil, and once it is warm, add the agar. Stir sporadically with a wooden spoon for 5 to 10 minutes until the agar is completely dissolved. Remove from heat and let cool (it can be lukewarm). Add the probiotic (just the powder) to the mixture and stir well with a wooden spoon (avoid metal).

Transfer the mixture to the glass jar and close with a tea towel and rubber band. Check after 48 hours. It should be slightly sour. Remove the tea towel and close with the regular lid.

Refrigerate for 2 hours and then process with the vanilla extract and agave. Make it creamy, and add the lemon at the end.

NUTRITIONAL INFORMATION 200g serving (1 cup)		
	Amount per serving	%DV(*)
Energetic value	486kcal or 2,041kJ	24
Carbohydrates	23g	8
Proteins	4g	5
Total fat	42g	76
Saturated fat	37g	168
Trans fats	-	**
Dietary fiber	4g	16
Sodium	31 mg	1

* % Daily Reference Values based on a 2000 kcal or 8400 kJ diet. Your daily values may be higher or lower depending on your energy needs.
** DV not established.

Peanut Butter Cookie
Yield: 3 servings
Preparation time: 20 minutes

Ingredients

- 1 egg
- 2 tablespoons of peanut butter
- 2 tablespoons of natural sweetener
- 2 tablespoons of unsweetened grated coconut
- 1 tablespoon of coconut flour

Preparation method

In a bowl, combine all the ingredients and mix well until a homogeneous dough forms.

Line a pan with aluminum and bake for 15 minutes.

NUTRITIONAL INFORMATION		
30g serving (1/2 unit)		
	Amount per serving	%DV(*)
Energetic value	73kcal or 307kJ	7
Carbohydrates	3g	1
Proteins	3g	4
Total fat	5.4g	10
Saturated fat	2.3g	10
Trans fats	-	**
Dietary fiber	1.5g	6
Sodium	10 mg	-

* % Daily Reference Values based on a 2000 kcal or 8400 kJ diet. Your daily values may be higher or lower depending on your energy needs.
** DV not established.

Carnivore Bread

Ingredients:

- 300g cooked and shredded chicken breast
- 5 eggs
- 1 small onion
- 2 tablespoons of grated cheese
- 1 tablespoon of butter
- 1 teaspoon baking soup

Preparation method

You can use any seasonings you like, such as sage, coriander, oregano, salt, etc. Butter can also be replaced with coconut oil or olive oil.

Place the chicken, cheese, butter, and yeast in a blender. Beat and stir with a spoon if you need to loosen the dough. If necessary, add a little of the water you used for cooking.

NUTRITIONAL INFORMATION		
90g serving (2 slices)		
	Amount per serving	%DV(*)
Energetic value	150kcal or 615kJ	7
Carbohydrates	2.1g	1
Proteins	17g	23
Total fat	8.1g	15
Saturated fat	2.9g	14
Trans fats	-	**
Dietary fiber	0.1g	-
Sodium	478 mg	20

* % Daily Reference Values based on a 2000 kcal or 8400 kJ diet. Your daily values may be higher or lower depending on your energy needs.
** DV not established.

Ketogenic Bread
Preparation Time: 10 minutes
Preparation: 35 minutes
Yield: 8 servings

Ingredients:

- 2 eggs
- 100g mozzarella
- 1 tablespoon of cream cheese (or cream)
- 1 cup of almond flour
- 1 tablespoon of chemical baking powder
- 1 tablespoon of apple cider vinegar

Preparation method

Grate the mozzarella or cut it into small pieces. Put it in a container, add the cottage cheese, and microwave until it melts, being careful not to burn it. Add the eggs and almond flour and mix well until the mixture is smooth. Add the yeast and then the apple cider vinegar. Mix gently. Transfer to a small greased or ungreased silicone cake tin. Bake in a preheated oven at 180°C for 30-35 minutes or until golden brown.

NUTRITIONAL INFORMATION		
45g serving (1 unit)		
	Amount per serving	%DV(*)
Energetic value	147kcal or 603kJ	7
Carbohydrates	4.1g	1
Proteins	7.8g	10
Total fat	11g	20
Saturated fat	2.8g	13
Trans fats	-	**
Dietary fiber	1.7g	7
Sodium	313 mg	13

* % Daily Reference Values based on a 2000 kcal or 8400 kJ diet. Your daily values may be higher or lower depending on your energy needs.
** DV not established.

Lunch

Avocado Sandwich
Yield: 1 serving
Preparation time: 15 minutes

Ingredients

- 2 slices of ketogenic bread
- Mashed avocado with nutritional yeast
- Spinach
- Cooked mini broccoli
- Sunflower sprouts
- Pink salt and black pepper to taste
- Bacon strips (marinated in coconut oil, paprika, salt and pepper, sautéed until crispy)

Preparation method

Assemble the sandwich however you like, starting with the mashed avocado.

NUTRITIONAL INFORMATION			
160g serving (1/2 unit)			
	Amount per serving	%DV(*)
Energetic value	229kcal or 939kJ	11
Carbohydrates	14g	5
Proteins	14g	19
Total fat	13g	24
Saturated fat	2.6g	12
Trans fats	-	**
Dietary fiber	7.5g	30
Sodium	449 mg	19

* % Daily Reference Values based on a 2000 kcal or 8400 kJ diet. Your daily values may be higher or lower depending on your energy needs.
** DV not established.

Fish in Mustard Sauce

Yield: 1 serving
Preparation time: 45 minutes

Ingredients

- 100g medium grouper fish fillet
- 1 teaspoon of crushed garlic
- 1 teaspoon of lemon juice
- 1 teaspoon of salt
- 1 teaspoon of extra virgin olive oil.

Sauce:

- 1 glass of cream
- 1 tablespoon of dark mustard
- ½ tablespoon of chopped fresh basil
- 1 pinch of salt.

How to make the sauce: mix all the ingredients, except the basil, in a deep bowl until the mixture is smooth. Keep in the fridge in a sealed container until ready to serve. Add the basil when serving.

Season the grouper with lemon, garlic, and salt and leave to marinate for between 15 and 20 minutes. Heat the non-stick frying pan with olive oil until it is very hot, then add the grouper. Brown the fish on both sides and remove it from the pan. Place the fish in a small ovenproof dish and set aside. When serving, heat the fish and add the hot sauce on top.

NUTRITIONAL INFORMATION			
150g serving (1/2 unit)			
	Amount per serving	%DV(*)
Energetic value	413kcal or 1,735kJ	21
Carbohydrates	16g	5
Proteins	13g	17
Total fat	33g	60
Saturated fat	13g	59
Trans fats	-	**
Dietary fiber	0.33g	1
Sodium	774 mg	32

* % Daily Reference Values based on a 2000 kcal or 8400 kJ diet. Your daily values may be higher or lower depending on your energy needs.
** DV not established.

Creamy Chicken Pancake

Yield: 1 serving

Preparation time: 15 minutes

Ingredients

- 1 egg white
- 1 egg
- 2 tablespoons of cottage cheese
- 1 pinch of turmeric
- 2 tablespoons of cream
- Fine herbs
- 80g chicken breast pre-seasoned with garlic, lemon and salt

Preparation method

Cook the chicken with some water and saffron; let the meat cool and shred it. Add the chicken, cream, and herbs and set aside.

Mix the egg, egg white, and cottage cheese in a bowl. Pour the batter into a hot frying pan greased with coconut oil, brown both sides, and turn off the heat. Fill the pancake with the chicken and fold it over.

| NUTRITIONAL INFORMATION ||
| 120g serving (1/2 unit) ||
Amount per serving	%DV(*)
Energetic value	280kcal or 1,176kJ	14
Carbohydrates	6.4g	2
Proteins	23g	31
Total fat	18g	33
Saturated fat	6.8g	31
Trans fats	-	**
Dietary fiber	3.2g	13
Sodium	428 mg	18

* % Daily Reference Values based on a 2000 kcal or 8400 kJ diet. Your daily values may be higher or lower depending on your energy needs.
** DV not established.

Mushroom Sauté
Yield: 3 servings
Preparation time: 20 minutes

Ingredients

- 10 fresh mushrooms
- 1 cup of fresh basil
- 10 mint leaves
- 2 tablespoons of olive oil
- 1 clove of garlic
- ½ cup of chopped walnuts

Preparation method
Clean the mushrooms with a damp cloth.
In a pan, heat the olive oil and garlic until golden brown.
Add the mushrooms and sauté well.
Finish with mint and basil leaves. Turn off the heat and sprinkle the walnuts.

NUTRITIONAL INFORMATION		
120g serving (1 unit)		
	Amount per serving	%DV(*)
Energetic value	218kcal or 916kJ	11
Carbohydrates	4.1g	1
Proteins	3.2g	4
Total fat	21g	38
Saturated fat	1.1g	5
Trans fats	-	**
Dietary fiber	2.2g	9
Sodium	71 mg	3

* % Daily Reference Values based on a 2000 kcal or 8400 kJ diet. Your daily values may be higher or lower depending on your energy needs.
** DV not established.

Mignon Stroganoff

Yield: 3 servings
Preparation time: 20 minutes

Ingredients

- Filet mignon in strips seasoned with salt and pepper
- ½ onion
- 3 cloves of garlic, chopped
- Olive oil drizzle
- 1 glass of milk of your choice
- 2 tablespoons of biomass
- 3 tablespoons of homemade tomato sauce
- Chopped chives

Preparation method

Sauté the onion and garlic in olive oil, add the tenderloin until golden brown, and set aside.

For the sauce, blend the milk with the biomass in a blender, then add the tomato sauce and stir until it thickens.

Pour the low-carb white sauce into the pan containing the tenderloin and serve with decorated spring onions.

NUTRITIONAL INFORMATION		
270g serving (1 unit)		
	Amount per serving	%DV(*)
Energetic value	300kcal or 1,260kJ	15
Carbohydrates	9.1g	3
Proteins	39g	52
Total fat	12g	22
Saturated fat	6.1g	28
Trans fats	-	**
Dietary fiber	1.1g	4
Sodium	181 mg	7

* % Daily Reference Values based on a 2000 kcal or 8400 kJ diet. Your daily values may be higher or lower depending on your energy needs.
** DV not established.

Crispy Snapper

Yield: 1 serving
Preparation time: 30 minutes

Ingredients

- 1 snapper fish fillet 150g
- Salt to taste
- Pink pepper to taste
- ½ rangpur
- 1 egg beaten with a pinch of salt and pepper
- ½ tablespoon of chia or passion fruit flour
- 2 tablespoons of crackling flour
- 2 tablespoons of grated Parmesan
- 1 drizzle of olive oil
- A piece of aluminum foil to line the pan

Preparation method
Preheat the oven to 200°C.
Line the baking tray with aluminum foil and grease with olive oil. Season the fish with salt, pepper, and lemon. Then, dip in the chia or passion fruit flour and the beaten egg. Finally, coat in the crackling flour mixed with grated Parmesan.

Bake for 20 minutes on one side and turn the fish over, baking for another 5 minutes.

Serve with lemon drops.

NUTRITIONAL INFORMATION		
200g serving (1 unit)		
	Amount per serving	%DV(*)
Energetic value	400kcal or 1,640kJ	20
Carbohydrates	7.6g	2
Proteins	41g	55
Total fat	40g	73
Saturated fat	12g	54
Trans fats	-	**
Dietary fiber	14g	56
Sodium	769 mg	32

* % Daily Reference Values based on a 2000 kcal or 8400 kJ diet. Your daily values may be higher or lower depending on your energy needs.
** DV not established.

Ceviche
Yield: 5 servings
Preparation time: 20 minutes

Ingredients

- 1 piece of finger pepper, seedless, finely chopped
- 2 tablespoons of chopped parsley
- 4 tablespoons of olive oil
- 3 units of juiced Tahiti lemon
- 500g St. Peter's fish or hake fillet, cubed
- Salt and pepper to taste

Preparation method

Mix all ingredients in a bowl and serve.

NUTRITIONAL INFORMATION		
110g serving (1 unit)		
	Amount per serving	%DV(*)
Energetic value	254kcal or 1,067kJ	13
Carbohydrates	3.8g	1
Proteins	26g	35
Total fat	15g	27
Saturated fat	1g	4
Trans fats	-	**
Dietary fiber	-	-
Sodium	128 mg	5
* % Daily Reference Values based on a 2000 kcal or 8400 kJ diet. Your daily values may be higher or lower depending on your energy needs. ** DV not established.		

Vegan Stroganoff
Yield: 2 servings
Preparation time: 40 minutes

Ingredients

- 2-3 cloves of garlic, chopped
- 1 tablespoon of vegetable oil
- 300g of sliced mushrooms
- 4 tablespoons of white wine (optional)
- 1 tablespoon of soy sauce
- 180ml of vegetable broth or water
- 180ml of cream

Preparation method

Heat the oil in a large frying pan, add the onion, and fry for about 5 minutes. Add the garlic and fry for another 1 minute. Add the mushrooms and fry on medium heat for about 5 minutes. Add the white wine (optional), vegetable broth, tamari (or soy sauce), and spice mix. Bring it to a boil. Add the cream and stir to dissolve.

Cook over medium-low heat for about 10 minutes until the sauce thickens. Taste and adjust seasonings to your preference. Add fresh thyme leaves. Enjoy with cauliflower rice.

NUTRITIONAL INFORMATION 300g serving (1 unit)		
	Amount per serving	%DV(*)
Energetic value	333kcal or 1,399kJ	17
Carbohydrates	19g	6
Proteins	5.7g	8
Total fat	26g	47
Saturated fat	9g	41
Trans fats	-	**
Dietary fiber	3.9g	15
Sodium	1,145 mg	48

* % Daily Reference Values based on a 2000 kcal or 8400 kJ diet. Your daily values may be higher or lower depending on your energy needs.
** DV not established.

Shrimp With Vegetables
Yield: 3 servings
Preparation time: 30 minutes

Ingredients

- 1 cup of cleaned shrimp
- ½ lemon squeezed
- ½ chopped pepper
- 1 cup of chopped chives
- 3 crushed garlic cloves
- 1 tablespoon of olive oil
- 1 cup of broccoli
- 1 cup of spinach

Preparation method

First, add the lemon juice and garlic to the shrimp to marinate and set aside. Sauté the peppers in a pan with a drizzle of olive oil until golden brown. Then add the prawns and cook. When it has taken on a more intense pink color, add the broccoli and spinach and cover the pan. Leave it on for 5 minutes and turn off. Add spring onions and serve with green leaves.

NUTRITIONAL INFORMATION 120g serving (1 unit)		
	Amount per serving	%DV(*)
Energetic value	97kcal or 407kJ	5
Carbohydrates	6.9g	2
Proteins	7.2g	10
Total fat	4.5g	8
Saturated fat	0.66g	3
Trans fats	-	**
Dietary fiber	3.9g	15
Sodium	98 mg	4
* % Daily Reference Values based on a 2000 kcal or 8400 kJ diet. Your daily values may be higher or lower depending on your energy needs. ** DV not established.		

Avocado Chicken Salad
Yield: 4 servings
Preparation time: 50 minutes

Ingredients

- 3 chicken breasts, bone-in and skinless
- 1 cup of dry white wine
- 1 cup of water
- 1 tablespoon of thyme leaves
- 2 tablespoons of Worcestershire sauce
- Salt and pepper to taste
- ½ diced avocado
- ¼ cup chopped fresh mint
- ¼ cup of olive oil
- Arugula leaves, lettuce, spinach and mini watercress

Preparation method

In a bowl, season the chicken with the wine, water, thyme, Worcestershire sauce, salt and pepper. Bake in a preheated oven (200°C), covered with aluminum foil, for 30 minutes or until cooked.

Remove the aluminum foil and bake, drizzling with the sauce from the baking sheet, for another 15 minutes or until golden brown. Let it warm up, and cut it into thin slices with a meat knife.

Mix the mint, olive oil, and salt in a bowl, and add the remaining stock to the roasting pan.

Arrange the rocket, lettuce, and spinach leaves on a platter.

Arrange the chicken slices on top. Spread the leaves and avocado, drizzle with the sauce and serve.

\	NUTRITIONAL INFORMATION 800g serving (1 unit)	
	Amount per serving	%DV(*)
Energetic value	380kcal or 1,596kJ	19
Carbohydrates	11g	4
Proteins	21g	28
Total fat	28g	51
Saturated fat	3.2g	14
Trans fats	-	**
Dietary fiber	7.6g	30
Sodium	146 mg	6
* % Daily Reference Values based on a 2000 kcal or 8400 kJ diet. Your daily values may be higher or lower depending on your energy needs. ** DV not established.		

Eggs with Mushrooms
Yield: 2 servings
Preparation time: 20 minutes

Ingredients

- 2 tablespoons of butter
- 250 g of mushrooms, sliced
- 4 eggs
- Salt and black pepper to taste

Preparation method

In a saucepan or frying pan, melt 1 tablespoon of butter and cook the mushrooms until they are soft and darker. Set aside. In a non-stick frying pan, melt the other tablespoon of butter and add the beaten eggs. Stir with a spoon and cook until firm but still soft. Serve the eggs and mushrooms while still warm.

NUTRITIONAL INFORMATION 245g serving (1 unit)		
	Amount per serving	%DV(*)
Energetic value	360kcal or 1,512kJ	18
Carbohydrates	7.6g	2
Proteins	15g	20
Total fat	30g	54
Saturated fat	14g	64
Trans fats	-	**
Dietary fiber	3g	12
Sodium	772 mg	32
* % Daily Reference Values based on a 2000 kcal or 8400 kJ diet. Your daily values may be higher or lower depending on your energy needs. ** DV not established.		

Vegetable Spaghetti with Basil Pesto
Yield: 3 servings
Preparation time: 15 minutes

Ingredients

- 4 medium carrots
- 2 cups of fresh basil
- ½ cup of roasted cashew nuts
- ½ cup of grated semi-hard cheese
- 2 garlic cloves
- ½ cup of extra virgin olive oil
- Lemon juice (½ lemon)
- 1 ice cube
- Salt and black pepper to taste

Preparation method

Cut the carrot into thin slices with a peeler.

Heat the frying pan with a drizzle of olive oil and lightly brown the garlic cloves. Sauté the sliced carrot until al dente. Season with a pinch of salt and black pepper.

Blend the olive oil, chestnuts, garlic, semi-cured cheese, and lemon juice in a blender. At the end, add the basil with a stone of ice (so it doesn't darken) and blend a little more. Then, all you have to do is assemble the dish (use a rim to shape it) and finish it with chopped cashew nuts.

NUTRITIONAL INFORMATION 230g serving (1 unit)		
	Amount per serving	%DV(*)
Energetic value	411kcal or 1,726kJ	20
Carbohydrates	19g	6
Proteins	14g	19g
Total fat	31g	56
Saturated fat	8.2g	37
Trans fats	-	**
Dietary fiber	6.8g	27
Sodium	181 mg	7
* % Daily Reference Values based on a 2000 kcal or 8400 kJ diet. Your daily values may be higher or lower depending on your energy needs. ** DV not established.		

Spinach Omelet Pizza
Yield: 1 serving
Preparation time: 30 minutes

Ingredients

- 2 free-range eggs
- 1 teaspoon of organic butter
- 1 cup of spinach (or green beans) previously sautéed in butter or olive oil (or steamed)

- ¼ small onion cut into thin slices (soak in water for 30 minutes)
- Extra virgin olive oil to taste
- Oregano to taste
- Basil to taste
- Cherry tomatoes cut into slices to taste
- Grated Parmesan (or cured) cheese to taste

Preparation method

Beat the eggs with a fork, add the salt, and set aside. In a frying pan, add the olive oil and a little butter. Pour in the beaten eggs.

Add the greens, tomatoes, onion, and lastly the cheese. Cover and leave on low heat for 3 minutes.

Finish with more oregano and basil.

NUTRITIONAL INFORMATION 220g serving (1 unit)		
	Amount per serving	%DV(*)
Energetic value	243kcal or 1,021kJ	12
Carbohydrates	10g	3
Proteins	17g	23
Total fat	15g	27
Saturated fat	6.5g	29
Trans fats	-	**
Dietary fiber	4.8g	19
Sodium	258 mg	11

* % Daily Reference Values based on a 2000 kcal or 8400 kJ diet. Your daily values may be higher or lower depending on your energy needs.
** DV not established.

Roasted Tilapia with Brazil Nuts
Yield: 4 servings
Preparation time: 55 minutes

Ingredients

- 4 tilapia fillets

- Lemon juice (½ lemon)
- Salt and pepper to taste
- 100g of chopped Brazil nuts
- 3 spoons of almond flour
- 1 tablespoon of chopped parsley
- 1 tablespoon of zero-sugar orange jelly
- 2 sweet potatoes cut into thick slices
- 2 onions cut into thick slices
- 100g cherry tomatoes

Preparation method

Season the tilapia with lemon, salt, and pepper. Mix the Brazil nuts, almond flour, parsley, and zero-sugar orange jelly in a bowl. Set aside.

Arrange the potatoes, onions, and tomatoes in a baking dish. Season with salt and pepper and drizzle with olive oil. Place the tilapia fillets, cover with the reserved mixture, then cover with aluminum foil and bake for 30 minutes.

Remove the aluminum foil and bake for 15 minutes or until golden brown.

NUTRITIONAL INFORMATION 300g serving (1 unit)		
	Amount per serving	%DV(*)
Energetic value	451kcal or 1,849kJ	22
Carbohydrates	24g	8
Proteins	28g	37
Total fat	27g	49
Saturated fat	6.0g	27
Trans fats	-	**
Dietary fiber	6.1g	28
Sodium	99 mg	4
* % Daily Reference Values based on a 2000 kcal or 8400 kJ diet. Your daily values may be higher or lower depending on your energy needs. ** DV not established.		

Dinner

Stuffed Chicken Burger

Yield: 7 servings
Preparation time: 30 minutes

Ingredients

- 2kg ground chicken breast
- 1 stalk of garlic, thinly sliced
- Mozzarella cheese slices
- Parsley
- Seasonings to taste
- Coconut oil (for greasing)

Preparation method

Mix everything except the cheese and put in the freezer for 10 minutes to make the mixture more consistent. To shape, place a layer of the seasoned chicken in the hamburger mold greased with coconut oil, then a slice of cheese and cover with some more chicken. Place the burger in a non-stick frying pan greased with a bit of coconut oil over low heat and brown both sides.

NUTRITIONAL INFORMATION 80g serving (1/4 of the unit)		
	Amount per serving	%DV(*)
Energetic value	140kcal or 588kJ	7
Carbohydrates	0.39g	-
Proteins	16g	21
Total fat	8.3g	15
Saturated fat	3.1g	14
Trans fats	-	**
Dietary fiber	-	-
Sodium	77 mg	3

* % Daily Reference Values based on a 2000 kcal or 8400 kJ diet. Your daily values may be higher or lower depending on your energy needs.
** DV not established.

Fit Soup
Yield: 3 servings
Preparation time: 40 minutes

Ingredients

- 1 large zucchini
- 2 small chayotes
- 1 clove of crushed garlic
- Parsley to taste
- 2 boneless chicken breasts

Preparation method

Start by preparing the vegetables, washing and cutting them. Sauté the garlic in a pan with a drizzle of olive oil. Add the vegetables and let them sauté. Add 1 and a half liters of water and boil over medium heat. Meanwhile, prepare the chicken breast, cooking it in the pressure cooker. When it is soft, turn it off, drain, and shred. When the vegetables are soft, wait for them to cool and blend in a blender with the broth until it becomes a soup. Return to the pan, add seasonings, and add the chicken. Mix well and serve. If you want, you can leave some vegetables in pieces.

NUTRITIONAL INFORMATION 760g serving (1 unit)		
	Amount per serving	%DV(*)
Energetic value	177kcal or 743kJ	9
Carbohydrates	6.8g	2
Proteins	19g	25
Total fat	8.2g	15
Saturated fat	2.3g	10
Trans fats	-	**
Dietary fiber	2.1g	8
Sodium	55 mg	2

* % Daily Reference Values based on a 2000 kcal or 8400 kJ diet. Your daily values may be higher or lower depending on your energy needs.
** DV not established.

Turkey Breast Basket

Yield: 6 servings
Preparation time: 20 minutes

Ingredients

- 6 slices of turkey breast
- 6 whole eggs
- Parsley and salt to taste
- Coconut oil (for greasing)

Preparation method

Grease cupcake tins with coconut oil, place a slice of turkey breast in each tin, break an egg on top of each slice, and sprinkle the seasoning. Place in the oven and turn it off as soon as the egg is cooked (to your taste).

NUTRITIONAL INFORMATION 74g serving (1 unit)		
	Amount per serving	%DV(*)
Energetic value	125kcal or 525kJ	6
Carbohydrates	1.4g	-
Proteins	14g	19
Total fat	6.8g	12
Saturated fat	1.9g	9
Trans fats	-	**
Dietary fiber	0.6g	2
Sodium	300 mg	12
* % Daily Reference Values based on a 2000 kcal or 8400 kJ diet. Your daily values may be higher or lower depending on your energy needs. ** DV not established.		

Zucchini Spaghetti

Yield: 2 servings
Preparation time: 30 minutes

Ingredients

- 1kg of Zucchini

- 1 tablespoon of minced garlic
- Salt and ground black pepper to taste
- 1 drizzle of olive oil
- 30g of basil leaves

Preparation method

Cut the zucchini into thin strips with a vegetable slicer so that they are in the shape of spaghetti and set aside. Over medium heat, sauté the garlic in a pan without letting it brown. Add 1 kg of ground knuckle steak and let it brown, then add 200 ml of hot water and let the excess water reduce. Adjust the seasoning with salt and ground black pepper to taste. Turn off the heat and set aside.

Heat 1 drizzle of olive oil in a frying pan and add the meat, zucchini spaghetti and mix. Turn off the heat and then serve on a plate, finishing with grated parmesan cheese, basil leaves, and olive oil to taste.

NUTRITIONAL INFORMATION 500g serving (1 unit)		
	Amount per serving	%DV(*)
Energetic value	188kcal or 790kJ	9
Carbohydrates	42g	14
Proteins	3.8g	5
Total fat	0.57g	1
Saturated fat	-	-
Trans fats	-	**
Dietary fiber	14g	56
Sodium	0.37 mg	-
* % Daily Reference Values based on a 2000 kcal or 8400 kJ diet. Your daily values may be higher or lower depending on your energy needs. ** DV not established.		

Cauliflower Cream
Yield: 3 servings
Preparation time: 30 minutes

Ingredients

- 4 cups of boiling water

- 500g of cauliflower in florets
- 10 unpeeled garlic cloves, cut in half
- Salt and black pepper
- 50g of grated Parmesan (plus more for sprinkling)

Preparation method

Bring the water with the cauliflower and garlic to a boil, with the pan covered, until softened (about 10 minutes).

Transfer the mixture to the blender glass, add salt, black pepper to taste, and Parmesan. Blend until smooth. Serve immediately, sprinkled with Parmesan and with chives or parsley to taste.

| NUTRITIONAL INFORMATION |||
| 320g serving (1 unit) |||
	Amount per serving	%DV(*)
Energetic value	145kcal or 609kJ	7
Carbohydrates	11g	4
Proteins	12g	16
Total fat	5.9g	11
Saturated fat	3.3g	15
Trans fats	-	**
Dietary fiber	4.7g	19
Sodium	250 mg	10

* % Daily Reference Values based on a 2000 kcal or 8400 kJ diet. Your daily values may be higher or lower depending on your energy needs.
** DV not established.

Carreteiro Cauliflower Rice
Yield: 5 servings
Preparation time: 50 minutes

Ingredients

- 1 head of cauliflower
- 1kg of dried meat
- 1 spoon of green scent
- 2 crushed garlic cloves
- 6 tablespoons of olive oil
- Salt to taste

Preparation method

Pass the raw cauliflower through a food processor (or blender) until it is about the size of rice grains (about 2 minutes).

Once processed, sauté with 1 tablespoon of olive oil for 3 minutes, turn off the heat and set aside.

Desalt the dried meat for 12 hours, then cook it until tender. Remove the water from the pan and shred it. Add the olive oil and brown the garlic in a pan, then add the shredded meat. Sauté everything until golden brown. Add the cauliflower rice (already made) and the green smell. Turn off the heat and stir well until smooth.

NUTRITIONAL INFORMATION 150g serving (1/2 unit)		
	Amount per serving	%DV(*)
Energetic value	389kcal or 1,634kJ	19
Carbohydrates	3.9g	1
Proteins	28g	37
Total fat	29g	53
Saturated fat	12g	54
Trans fats	-	**
Dietary fiber	1.9g	8
Sodium	442 mg	18

* % Daily Reference Values based on a 2000 kcal or 8400 kJ diet. Your daily values may be higher or lower depending on your energy needs.
** DV not established.

Souffle of Broccoli
Yield: 4 servings
Preparation time: 60 minutes

Ingredients

- 350g of chopped broccoli
- 1/3 cup of rice flour
- 1 ½ cups of skimmed milk
- 1/3 cup of low-calorie cream

- 1 tablespoon of lemon zest
- ¾ teaspoon of salt
- 3 egg yolks, sifted (without the skin)
- 1 clove of minced garlic
- 6 egg whites
- Olive oil spray
- Grated cheese for sprinkling

Preparation method

Cook the broccoli for about 4 minutes, or until tender, and set aside.

Place the flour and milk in a pan and stir well until it boils. Reduce heat and add cream, lemon zest, salt, egg yolks, and garlic. Cook for 1 minute or until thickened, stirring constantly. Pour the mixture into a large bowl and add the broccoli. Beat the egg whites with a mixer at high speed until stiff peaks form. Gently mix the egg whites into the broccoli.

Place the mixture in a refractory, greased with olive oil, and sprinkle with cheese.

Place in the oven to bake for around 40 minutes. When it is browned, remove it to serve.

NUTRITIONAL INFORMATION		
200g serving (1 unit)		
	Amount per serving	%DV(*)
Energetic value	184kcal or 773kJ	9
Carbohydrates	17g	6
Proteins	13g	17
Total fat	7.1g	13
Saturated fat	2.8g	13
Trans fats	-	**
Dietary fiber	3.2g	13
Sodium	493 mg	20

* % Daily Reference Values based on a 2000 kcal or 8400 kJ diet. Your daily values may be higher or lower depending on your energy needs.
** DV not established.

Kibbeh Stuffed with Ricotta
Yield: 10 servings
Preparation time: 50 minutes

Ingredients

- 500g of kibbeh wheat
- 500g of ground knuckle steak
- 3 cups of boiling water
- 1 chopped onion
- 4 tablespoons of chopped mint
- Salt to taste
- 1 tablespoon of butter

Filling

- 400g of mashed ricotta
- 8 tablespoons of chopped mint
- 1 cup of Brazil nuts
- 1 tablespoon of olive oil for brushing

Preparation method

Leave the wheat to soak in water for approximately 30 minutes and then remove excess water.

Add the onion, mint, salt, and butter and mix well. Add the meat and mix until it becomes a homogeneous paste.

Place the dough between two plastic wraps to freeze and roll out with a rolling pin. Remove the plastic and cut the dough in half.

On one of the parts, spread the filling. Place the other part over the filling. Then, cut the dough and shape it with your hands, sealing the sides well.

Place them on a baking sheet, brush with olive oil, and bake in a preheated 180°C oven until golden brown.

| NUTRITIONAL INFORMATION ||||
| 100g serving (1/2 unit) ||||
	Amount per serving	%DV(*)
Energetic value	225kcal or 945kJ	11
Carbohydrates	22g	7
Proteins	12g	16
Total fat	9.9g	18
Saturated fat	3.5g	16
Trans fats	-	**
Dietary fiber	5.7g	23
Sodium	40 mg	1
* % Daily Reference Values based on a 2000 kcal or 8400 kJ diet. Your daily values may be higher or lower depending on your energy needs. ** DV not established.			

Spinach Cream

Yield: 4 servings
Preparation time: 10 minutes

Ingredients

- ½ bunch of washed spinach
- 1 tablespoon of margarine
- 1 chopped small onion
- Garlic to taste
- 2 tablespoons of cornstarch
- ½ liter of milk
- 1 can of cream
- 100 g of grated Parmesan

Preparation method

Boil the spinach leaves in salted water for approximately 4 minutes. Drain, squeeze, and chop them.

Heat the margarine, sauté the onion and garlic in a pan, and add the spinach.

Add the cornstarch diluted in the milk and stir until it thickens. Turn off the heat, and mix the cream and grated cheese.

NUTRITIONAL INFORMATION		
280g serving (1 unit)		
	Amount per serving	%DV(*)
Energetic value	464kcal or 1,949kJ	23
Carbohydrates	25g	8
Proteins	19g	25
Total fat	32g	58
Saturated fat	15g	68
Trans fats	-	**
Dietary fiber	1.8g	7
Sodium	606 mg	25
* % Daily Reference Values based on a 2000 kcal or 8400 kJ diet. Your daily values may be higher or lower depending on your energy needs. ** DV not established.		

Mexican-style Fried Scallops
Yield: 4 servings
Preparation time: 15 minutes

Ingredients

- 2 tablespoons of butter
- 2 tablespoons of olive oil
- 200g of scallops without the shell
- 1 onion
- 2 garlic cloves
- 1 handful of coriander
- 1 handful of chives
- ½ seedless jalapeno pepper
- Lemon juice (½ lemon)
- Salt to taste

Preparation method
Season the scallops with salt and set aside.
Chop and peel the garlic cloves, onion, coriander, chives and pepper. Set aside.

In a frying pan, add the butter and heat it. Let the butter heat up well. Then, add the scallops to be seared. Seal both sides of the scallops and remove them from the pan.

Add the olive oil to the pan to use the butter. Also, add the garlic, onion and pepper. Season with salt and let it cook for a few moments. Add the coriander and chives.

Add the lemon juice and return the scallops to the pan. Remove the pan from the heat after 3 minutes; it will be ready to serve.

NUTRITIONAL INFORMATION 100g serving (1 unit)		
	Amount per serving	%DV(*)
Energetic value	223kcal or 937kJ	11
Carbohydrates	7.9g	3
Proteins	9.6g	13
Total fat	17g	31
Saturated fat	4.7g	21
Trans fats	-	**
Dietary fiber	0.82g	3
Sodium	245 mg	10
* % Daily Reference Values based on a 2000 kcal or 8400 kJ diet. Your daily values may be higher or lower depending on your energy needs. ** DV not established.		

Bone Broth to Boost Immunity
Yield: 6 servings
Preparation time: 4 hours and 50 minutes

Ingredients

- 1 kg of bones (with marrow), you can have the meat along with it. If possible, put feet, joints, and viscera together.
- Salt, garlic, turmeric, black pepper, marjoram and oregano to taste
- 3 tablespoons of apple cider vinegar
- Fill 2/3 of the pan with water

Preparation method

Cook for 3 hours for beef or 2 hours for chicken in the pressure cooker. Stop halfway through to top up with water if your pressure cooker is small (3 or 4 liters), or go straight to the end if your pressure cooker is large (6 or 7 liters). Strain and serve.

NUTRITIONAL INFORMATION		
250ml serving (1 deep plate)		
	Amount per serving	%DV(*)
Energetic value	494kcal or 2,075kJ	25
Carbohydrates	-	-
Proteins	4.2g	6
Total fat	53g	96
Saturated fat	-	-
Trans fats	-	**
Dietary fiber	-	-
Sodium	-	-
* % Daily Reference Values based on a 2000 kcal or 8400 kJ diet. Your daily values may be higher or lower depending on your energy needs. ** DV not established.		

Chicken Soufflé
Yield: 3 servings
Preparation time: 30 minutes

Ingredients

- 100 g of shredded chicken
- 1 egg
- 1 egg white
- Parsley
- Basil
- 1 tablespoon of tomato cubes
- 1 tablespoon of cottage cheese
- Parmesan to finish (optional)

Preparation method
Preheat the oven to 200°c.
Beat the egg and white until they are uniform.
Put the chicken mixed with the seasonings and tomatoes in a heatproof dish. Pour the egg mixture over the top. Finish with cottage cheese and Parmesan.

Bake for 20 minutes or until golden brown.

NUTRITIONAL INFORMATION			
70g serving (1 unit)			
	Amount per serving	%DV(*)
Energetic value	101kcal or 424kJ	5
Carbohydrates	0.97g	-
Proteins	12g	16
Total fat	5.5g	10
Saturated fat	1.4g	6
Trans fats	-	**
Dietary fiber	-	-
Sodium	68 mg	3

* % Daily Reference Values based on a 2000 kcal or 8400 kJ diet. Your daily values may be higher or lower depending on your energy needs.
** DV not established.

Scrambled Eggs with Leek and Parmesan

Yield: 2 servings

Preparation time: 10 minutes

Ingredients

- 2 whole eggs
- 1 tablespoon of full of grated Parmesan
- 1 tablespoon of skimmed milk
- 1 cup of sliced leeks
- Salt and pepper to taste

Preparation method

Cut the leek into slices in the white part. Beat the eggs with the milk, add the leek, and season with salt and pepper. Heat a non-stick frying pan with a bit of olive oil or light butter and pour in the mixture. Let it cook, stirring constantly.

| NUTRITIONAL INFORMATION |||
| 110g serving (1 unit) |||
	Amount per serving	%DV(*)
Energetic value	107kcal or 448kJ	5
Carbohydrates	3.9g	1
Proteins	8.6g	11
Total fat	6.3g	11
Saturated fat	2.4g	11
Trans fats	-	**
Dietary fiber	1.1g	4
Sodium	117 mg	5

* % Daily Reference Values based on a 2000 kcal or 8400 kJ diet. Your daily values may be higher or lower depending on your energy needs.
** DV not established.

Omelet of the Gods

Yield: 1 serving
Preparation time: 15 minutes

Ingredients

- 2 eggs
- 1 cup of grated semi-cured Minas cheese
- ¼ chopped onion
- ½ chopped tomato
- ½ cup of spinach
- Salt, black pepper, and olive oil to taste

Preparation method

Heat the oil in a frying pan, add the onion, tomato, spinach, and sauté—season with salt and pepper and set aside.

In a bowl, break the eggs and season with salt and pepper. Stir with a whisk or fork.

In the same frying pan where you prepared the vegetables, add more olive oil, heat it up, and add the eggs. Mix the contents of the pan a little with a fork so that it covers the surface of the pan, and as soon as you notice that the bottom is starting to brown and come away from the pan, turn off the heat, allowing the filling to become creamy.

Add the sautéed vegetables and cheese to this creamy part, pulling the sides of the omelet together to form a small border so that the contents of the filling don't get lost. Turn the heat back on and slowly close the omelet. Serve immediately to enjoy the recipe's creamy filling.

NUTRITIONAL INFORMATION 145g serving (1/2 unit)		
	Amount per serving	%DV(*)
Energetic value	260kcal or 1,091kJ	13
Carbohydrates	5.2g	2
Proteins	17g	23
Total fat	19g	34
Saturated fat	10g	45
Trans fats	-	**
Dietary fiber	1.4g	6
Sodium	315 mg	13
* % Daily Reference Values based on a 2000 kcal or 8400 kJ diet. Your daily values may be higher or lower depending on your energy needs. ** DV not established.		

Avocado Pate with Chicken
Yield: 5 servings
Preparation time: 5 minutes

Ingredients

- 2 tablespoons of avocado
- 1 lemon squeezed
- Mint leaves to taste
- ½ chopped tomato
- 1 tablespoon of shredded chicken

Preparation method

Clean the vegetables. Chop the tomatoes and mix with the avocado to form a smooth paste. Add the lemon and leave for 10 minutes to concentrate the flavor. Add the chicken and mix once more.

NUTRITIONAL INFORMATION			
60g serving (3 tablespoons)			
	Amount per serving	%DV(*)
Energetic value	58kcal or 245kJ	3
Carbohydrates	2.8g	1
Proteins	3.5g	5
Total fat	3.7g	7
Saturated fat	0.76g	3
Trans fats	-	**
Dietary fiber	2g	8
Sodium	3.7 mg	-
* % Daily Reference Values based on a 2000 kcal or 8400 kJ diet. Your daily values may be higher or lower depending on your energy needs. ** DV not established.			

Pancake with Chicken
Yield: 3 servings
Preparation time: 10 minutes

Ingredients

- 4 units of egg white
- 1 tablespoon of oat bran
- 1 pinch of salt and black pepper
- 5 tablespoons of cooked and shredded chicken (or sautéed ground beef)
- 2 tablespoons of tomato sauce
- 1 tablespoon of semi-cured cheese

Preparation method

Beat the egg whites with the oat bran, salt and pepper. Prepare the pancake in a medium non-stick frying pan greased with 1 drizzle of olive oil—Brown on both sides and stuff with shredded chicken (or ground beef). Serve with the sauce and grated cheese.

NUTRITIONAL INFORMATION		
145g serving (1 unit)		
	Amount per serving	%DV(*)
Energetic value	133kcal or 559kJ	7
Carbohydrates	5.1g	2
Proteins	20g	27
Total fat	3.6g	7
Saturated fat	1.6g	7
Trans fats	-	**
Dietary fiber	1.1g	4
Sodium	283 mg	12

* % Daily Reference Values based on a 2000 kcal or 8400 kJ diet. Your daily values may be higher or lower depending on your energy needs.
** DV not established.

Zucchini Ravioli
Yield: 1 serving
Preparation time: 20 minutes

Ingredients

- 4 slices of zucchini (cut lengthwise) grilled in a non-stick frying pan with 1 drizzle of olive oil
- 1 chicken fillet cooked with seasonings of your choice and shredded
- 1 slice of cheese of your choice, chopped
- Homemade Tomato Sauce

Preparation method

Place the zucchini slices in a cross shape. Place the chicken and cheese in the center. Fold. Add the sauce and bake at 180°C for 15 minutes.

NUTRITIONAL INFORMATION		
500g serving (1 unit)		
	Amount per serving	%DV(*)
Energetic value	413kcal or 1,735kJ	21
Carbohydrates	32g	11
Proteins	33g	44

Total fat	17g	31
Saturated fat	7.7g	35
Trans fats	-	**
Dietary fiber	6.8g	27
Sodium	233 mg	10

* % Daily Reference Values based on a 2000 kcal or 8400 kJ diet. Your daily values may be higher or lower depending on your energy needs.
** DV not established.

Spinach Quiche with Almond Flour
Yield: 8 servings
Preparation time: 40 minutes

Ingredients

- ½ cup of almond flour
- ¼ cup of olive oil (add a little more if the dough is crumbly)
- 1 pinch of salt

Filling

- 1 bunch of washed spinach (filling)
- 4 eggs
- ¼ cup of fresh cream (or vegetable milk: chestnut, almond, oat)
- 1 teaspoon of chemical yeast
- 1 cup of grated parmesan cheese

Preparation method

Mix all the ingredients for the dough (almond flour, olive oil, and salt) in a bowl until it forms a dough. Line the bottom and sides of a medium-sized removable-rimmed baking tin. Bake in a preheated oven at 180 °C for 15 minutes. Set aside.

Sauté the spinach with 1 drizzle of olive oil for 2 minutes. Add the eggs, cream, yeast, and Parmesan, mix well, and pour over the dough. Bake for another 20 minutes or until completely baked (or test with a toothpick).

| NUTRITIONAL INFORMATION |||
| 80g serving (1 unit) |||
	Amount per serving	%DV(*)
Energetic value	204kcal or 857kJ	10
Carbohydrates	5.1g	2
Proteins	10g	13
Total fat	16g	29
Saturated fat	3.8g	17
Trans fats	-	**
Dietary fiber	2.3g	9
Sodium	285 mg	12

* % Daily Reference Values based on a 2000 kcal or 8400 kJ diet. Your daily values may be higher or lower depending on your energy needs.
** DV not established.

Zucchini Cream with Chicken

Yield: 4 servings
Preparation time: 20 minutes

Ingredients

- 2 zucchinis
- 2 tablespoons of cream cheese
- 1 tablespoon of cream
- 50 grams grated Parmesan
- ½ shredded chicken breast
- 2 garlic cloves
- Salt and black pepper
- Butter for frying

Preparation method

Cover the zucchini cut into large pieces with water in a saucepan and cook until soft—season with a bit of salt and black pepper.

Drain the zucchini and transfer them to a blender or processor. Blend well until it turns into a puree. Set aside the cooking water to adjust the soup's texture at the end. Transfer the puree to a saucepan.

To make the shredded chicken, use this recipe's "ninja" technique. When I make it, I prepare an extra amount and store frozen portions in jars.

Fry the shredded chicken with the crushed garlic cloves and a spoonful of butter—season with a bit of salt and pepper.

Add the chicken, grated Parmesan cheese, cream cheese, and cream (or cream). Mix well and let it cook a little to incorporate the flavors.

NUTRITIONAL INFORMATION		
225g serving (1 unit)		
	Amount per serving	%DV(*)
Energetic value	200kcal or 840kJ	10
Carbohydrates	7g	2
Proteins	16g	21
Total fat	12g	22
Saturated fat	6.2g	28
Trans fats	-	**
Dietary fiber	1.8g	7
Sodium	305 mg	13

* % Daily Reference Values based on a 2000 kcal or 8400 kJ diet. Your daily values may be higher or lower depending on your energy needs.
** DV not established.

Ketogenic chicken pizza

On a pizza, we must worry about the dough and the toppings. There are several strategies for adapting pasta to the ketogenic diet, including cauliflower, broccoli, chicken, and other flours.

Preparation: 5 minutes
Preparation: 35 minutes
Yield: 8 servings

Ingredients

- 450g of ground or shredded chicken
- 1 egg
- 1 cup of fresh grated cheese (80g)
- Salt to taste

- Optional filling

Preparation method

Place the ground chicken meat in a bowl, then add the egg, cheese, salt, and seasoning to taste. Mix well with your hands until the dough is smooth. Line a pizza pan with baking paper. Transfer this mixture and gently spread the dough into a pizza disc, not too thick or thin. Bake in a preheated oven at 180° C for about 20 to 25 minutes. The dough is ready when it is golden brown. Remove the dough from the oven, add your chosen filling, and return to the oven for another 10 minutes.

NUTRITIONAL INFORMATION 72g serving (1 slice)		
	Amount per serving	%DV(*)
Energetic value	126kcal or 517kJ	6
Carbohydrates	0.6g	-
Proteins	18g	24
Total fat	5.7g	10
Saturated fat	1.9g	9
Trans fats	-	**
Dietary fiber	-	-
Sodium	261 mg	11

* % Daily Reference Values based on a 2000 kcal or 8400 kJ diet. Your daily values may be higher or lower depending on your energy needs.
** DV not established.

Keto Cauliflower Pizza
Preparation: 35 minutes
Yield: 8 servings

Ingredients

- 1 medium or small cauliflower
- ½ cup of fresh mozzarella or Parmesan
- ½ cup of grated Parmesan
- Salt and seasonings to taste
- 1 small egg

Preparation method

Remove the outer leaves from the cauliflower. Wash and dry them well. Place all of the cauliflower into a food processor or blender. Blend in pulse mode until it reaches a flour-like consistency. Transfer the crushed cauliflower to a preheated pan and sauté over low heat for 5 minutes. Transfer to a clean cloth and squeeze well until all remaining liquid is removed. Transfer to another container. Add the egg, cheese, optional seasonings, and salt. Mix well, kneading with your hands. Grease a mold, preferably non-stick. Spread the dough using your hands, making it very smooth. If your dough is thick, it will need more baking time. Make it approximately 1cm wide. Bake in a preheated oven at 180° degrees for 20 minutes.

Meanwhile, prepare the filling. Remove the pizza from the oven, spread with tomato sauce, and add the desired toppings. Return to the oven and let it bake at 180°C until the filling is ready.

| NUTRITIONAL INFORMATION |||
| 60g serving (1 slice) |||
	Amount per serving	%DV(*)
Energetic value	56kcal or 231kJ	3
Carbohydrates	0.9g	-
Proteins	4.9g	6
Total fat	3.7g	7
Saturated fat	2.1g	9
Trans fats	-	**
Dietary fiber	0.2g	1
Sodium	158 mg	6
* % Daily Reference Values based on a 2000 kcal or 8400 kJ diet. Your daily values may be higher or lower depending on your energy needs.		
** DV not established.		

Desserts

Ketogenic yogurt and cream cheese

Yogurt is a living food. Fermentation transforms sugar and carbohydrates so that the food can enter the ketogenic diet. However, most industrialized yogurts do not consist of original yogurt but a mixture containing honey, starch, and other added sugars. After much research in São Paulo, I found only one brand with proportions closer to the ketogenic diet. I think the difficulty is the same everywhere. There is no point in choosing just any yogurt in the supermarket. You need to find the original or make your own to use yogurt.

In the ideal homemade yogurt, we use raw milk straight from the cow. The amount of fats is much higher, and you can also opt for cows or goats that have A2 casein, avoiding casein allergy problems. Raw milk contains noticeably more fat than industrialized whole milk and many more probiotic microorganisms than supermarket milk or yogurt. To prepare this yogurt, you will use a yogurt maker, milk, and a yogurt pot as an activator, which can be replaced with a packet of probiotic starter cultures of your choice. To control and reduce the amount of sugars and carbohydrates, the variable we modify is the fermentation time. Increase the fermentation time as much as possible until it is firm. If the recommended time was 6 hours, we suggest 12 hours in summer or even 18 hours in winter. Remember that fermentation is faster at higher temperatures. Once this is done, put the yogurt in the fridge. The next step is desiccation: take a pot and a clean tea towel. Fix the tea towel to the mouth of the pot with a rubber band. Remove your finished yogurt from the refrigerator and place it on a tea towel. Place the lid on the pot so harmful bacteria do not colonize the food. Take it back to the fridge to drain for 18 hours. After waiting, your Greek yogurt will be ready: the paste remains on the kitchen towel. Remove this yogurt paste with a spoon, place it in a jar, and leave it in the refrigerator.

When you taste it, you'll notice that Greek yogurt is sourer, as the sugar has almost all gone during fermentation. It should be a creamy paste. If it's runny, it's been too long. The original cream cheese is nothing more than ketogenic Greek yogurt that has been drained for longer and added spices. To complete the ketogenic homemade cream cheese, beat the cream with some spices of your choice and salt. Oregano, parsley, and garlic will add a special touch.

Protein Avocado
Yield: 3 servings
Preparation time: 5 minutes

Ingredients

- 1 small avocado
- ½ lemon
- 1 scoop of vanilla whey protein
- ½ glass of water
- 1 tablespoon of grated coconut for sprinkling

Preparation method

Mix all the ingredients in a blender until smooth—place in the refrigerator for at least an hour. When serving, sprinkle the freshly grated coconut on top.

| NUTRITIONAL INFORMATION |||
| 60g serving (3 tablespoons) |||
	Amount per serving	%DV(*)
Energetic value	81kcal or 340kJ	4
Carbohydrates	3.3g	1
Proteins	2.1g	3
Total fat	6.6g	12
Saturated fat	1.8g	8
Trans fats	-	**
Dietary fiber	3g	12
Sodium	4.2 mg	-

* % Daily Reference Values based on a 2000 kcal or 8400 kJ diet. Your daily values may be higher or lower depending on your energy needs.
** DV not established.

Peanut Butter Cookie
Yield: 3 servings
Preparation time: 20 minutes

Ingredients

- 1 egg
- 2 tablespoons of peanut butter
- 2 tablespoons of natural sweetener
- 2 tablespoons of unsweetened grated coconut
- 1 tablespoon of coconut flour

Preparation method

In a bowl, combine all the ingredients and mix well until a homogeneous dough forms. Line a pan with aluminum and bake for 15 minutes.

NUTRITIONAL INFORMATION			
30g serving (1/2 unit)			
	Amount per serving		%DV(*)
Energetic value	73kcal or 307kJ		7
Carbohydrates	3g		1
Proteins	3g		4
Total fat	5.4g		10
Saturated fat	2.3g		10
Trans fats	-		**
Dietary fiber	1.5g		6
Sodium	10 mg		-
* % Daily Reference Values based on a 2000 kcal or 8400 kJ diet. Your daily values may be higher or lower depending on your energy needs. ** DV not established.			

Homemade Peanut Butter

Yield: 2 servings

Preparation time: 20 minutes

Ingredients

- 1 kg of roasted skinless peanuts
- 2 tablespoons of coconut oil
- ½ cup of xylitol

Preparation method

Place the peanuts in a baking dish and bake in an oven at 180°C for 15 minutes to warm them slightly.

Put the very hot peanuts in a food processor and blend until they are small, moist pieces.

Add the coconut oil xylitol and beat again until it becomes creamy. This will take a while, so take it easy, keep beating, and, if necessary, stop so the equipment can rest.

Place in a clean jar with a lid and refrigerate.

NUTRITIONAL INFORMATION			
10g serving (1 tablespoon)			
	Amount per serving		%DV(*)
Energetic value	63kcal or 258kJ		3
Carbohydrates	2.6g		1
Proteins	2.7g		4
Total fat	4.6g		8
Saturated fat	1.0g		4
Trans fats	-		**
Dietary fiber	0.4g		2
Sodium	0.9 mg		-

* % Daily Reference Values based on a 2000 kcal or 8400 kJ diet. Your daily values may be higher or lower depending on your energy needs.
** DV not established.

Avocado Ice Cream with Matcha

Yield: 900ml
Preparation time: 3 hours and 10 minutes

Ingredients

- 2 large ripe avocados
- Lemon juice (½ lemon)
- 2 level teaspoons of organic matcha
- 1 tablespoon of xylitol honey
- 1 teaspoon of ginger powder (optional)
- ¼ teaspoon of sea salt
- ½ cup of chilled coconut milk
- 1 cup of raw cashew nuts (hydrated for at least 4 hours - discard the water)
- ½ ripe banana
- ¼ cup xylitol

Preparation method

Blend all ingredients until you form a smooth and homogeneous cream.

Place in the freezer for at least 3 hours. Serve with cocoa nibs[xxxvii] *or dark chocolate chips.*

NUTRITIONAL INFORMATION 60g serving (1 scoop of ice cream)		
	Amount per serving	%DV(*)
Energetic value	119kcal or 488kJ	6
Carbohydrates	7.8g	3
Proteins	1.6g	2
Total fat	9.1g	16
Saturated fat	2.1g	9
Trans fats	-	**
Dietary fiber	1.7g	7
Sodium	41 mg	2
* % Daily Reference Values based on a 2000 kcal or 8400 kJ diet. Your daily values may be higher or lower depending on your energy needs. ** DV not established.		

Pomegranate Gelato
Yield: 5 servings
Preparation time: 1 hour and 10 minutes

Ingredients

- 2 tablespoons of rice milk
- 2 tablespoons of pomegranate seeds
- 1 frozen and chopped banana
- 2 tablespoons of vanilla whey
- 1 tablespoon of rolled oats

Preparation method
Separate the pomegranate seeds.
Add the rest of the ingredients to the blender and blend until smooth.

[xxxvii] Chocolate in its purest form is the seeds of the so-called cocoa bean. After roasting them, they are peeled and crushed. It is a bitter food that has the intense flavor of a chocolate with a high cocoa content. This is the raw material for making quality dark chocolate.

Spread the cream in a baking dish or individual dessert jars. Add the pomegranate seeds and chill in the freezer for at least an hour.

NUTRITIONAL INFORMATION 60g serving (1 scoop of ice cream)			
	Amount per serving	%DV(*)
Energetic value	71kcal or 298kJ	4
Carbohydrates	8.6g	3
Proteins	6.8g	9
Total fat	1g	2
Saturated fat	-	-
Trans fats	-	**
Dietary fiber	0.73g	3
Sodium	20 mg	1
* % Daily Reference Values based on a 2000 kcal or 8400 kJ diet. Your daily values may be higher or lower depending on your energy needs. ** DV not established.			

Red Fruit Ice Cream
Yield: 4 servings
Preparation time: 3 hours and 30 minutes

Ingredients

- 1 cup of green banana biomass
- 2 tablespoons of light coconut milk
- 1 cup of frozen strawberries, blueberries and cranberries

Preparation method

Heat the fruits with the coconut milk until you create a homogeneous mixture.

Add the biomass and mix well. It will be airy. Add another spoonful of coconut milk if you want a creamier ice cream.

Wait for it to cool and put it in the freezer.

NUTRITIONAL INFORMATION			
60g serving (1 scoop of ice cream)			
	Amount per serving	%DV(*)
Energetic value	45kcal or 189kJ	2
Carbohydrates	7.6g	2
Proteins	0.59g	1
Total fat	1.4g	2
Saturated fat	-	-
Trans fats	-	**
Dietary fiber	1.4g	6
Sodium	1.3 mg	-

* % Daily Reference Values based on a 2000 kcal or 8400 kJ diet. Your daily values may be higher or lower depending on your energy needs.
** DV not established.

Tropical Fruit Ice Cream

Yield: 4 servings

Preparation time: 3 hours and 30 minutes

Ingredients

- 1 cup of green banana biomass
- 2 tablespoons of light coconut milk
- 1 cup of frozen mango, tangerine and orange

Preparation method

Heat the fruits with the coconut milk until you create a homogeneous mixture.

Add the biomass and mix well. It will be airy. Add another spoonful of coconut milk if you want a creamier ice cream.

Wait for it to cool and put it in the freezer.

NUTRITIONAL INFORMATION			
60g serving (1 scoop of ice cream)			
	Amount per serving	%DV(*)
Energetic value	56kcal or 235kJ	3
Carbohydrates	10g	3
Proteins	0.73g	1
Total fat	1.5g	3
Saturated fat	-	-
Trans fats	-	**
Dietary fiber	2.2g	9
Sodium	1.6 mg	-
* % Daily Reference Values based on a 2000 kcal or 8400 kJ diet. Your daily values may be higher or lower depending on your energy needs. ** DV not established.			

Lactose-Free Avocado Ice Cream
Yield: 6 servings
Preparation time: 4 hours and 50 minutes

Ingredients

- 2 peeled and pitted avocados
- 1 cup of hot water
- ½ cup of culinary sweetener
- ½ cup of lactose-free low-fat natural yogurt
- ½ teaspoon of vanilla essence

Preparation method

Blend the avocado in a blender until creamy.

Mix the hot water and sweetener heat in a pan until completely dissolved.

Add the dissolved sweetener to the avocado and mix well. Freeze for 4 to 6 hours until firm, stirring every hour to break up the ice crystals. When it's firm, put the mixture, the yogurt, and the vanilla essence in a blender, blend until smooth, and place in the freezer.

NUTRITIONAL INFORMATION		
60g serving (1 scoop of ice cream)		
	Amount per serving	%DV(*)
Energetic value	73kcal or 306kJ	4
Carbohydrates	3.4g	1
Proteins	0.8g	1
Total fat	6.2g	11
Saturated fat	1.2g	5
Trans fats	-	**
Dietary fiber	3.2g	13
Sodium	23 mg	1
* % Daily Reference Values based on a 2000 kcal or 8400 kJ diet. Your daily values may be higher or lower depending on your energy needs. ** DV not established.		

Protein Chocolate Mousse
Yield: 900ml
Preparation time: 3 hours and 10 minutes

Ingredients

- 300g of 70% chocolate
- 9 egg whites
- 200ml of lactose-free cream
- 1 scoop of chocolate whey
- 2 tablespoons of xylitol

Preparation method

Melt the chocolate over a water bath, add the cream, mix until it forms a ganache, and wait for it to cool. Add the egg white gently, mixing from bottom to top, and add the xylitol and whey, mixing well. Place the dough in jars and let it freeze for 3 hours—yields 900ml of mousse.

| NUTRITIONAL INFORMATION |||
| 20g serving (1 tablespoon) |||
	Amount per serving	%DV(*)
Energetic value	50kcal or 205kJ	2
Carbohydrates	2.9g	1
Proteins	1.9g	2
Total fat	3.4g	6
Saturated fat	2.1g	9
Trans fats	-	**
Dietary fiber	0.6g	2
Sodium	13 mg	-
* % Daily Reference Values based on a 2000 kcal or 8400 kJ diet. Your daily values may be higher or lower depending on your energy needs. ** DV not established.		

Peanut Butter Pie
Yield: 6 servings
Preparation time: 40 minutes

Ingredients

- 1 cup of peanut butter
- ¼ cup xylitol coconut sugar
- 1/3 cup coconut flour
- ½ cup of melted coconut oil
- 100 grams of dark chocolate, 80% cocoa, chopped
- 2 tablespoons of peanut butter

Preparation method

Blend the peanut butter, sugar, flour, and coconut oil in a food processor until it forms a smooth paste.

Place the dough on a baking sheet lined with parchment paper and then put the contents in the freezer for about 20 minutes.

Melt the chocolate and add two tablespoons of peanut butter. Stir well.

Spread the contents over the base and return it to the freezer for another two hours.

Remove the pie and wait 10 to 15 minutes to serve.

| NUTRITIONAL INFORMATION |||
| 60g serving (1 unit) |||
	Amount per serving	%DV(*)
Energetic value	407kcal or 1,669kJ	20
Carbohydrates	13g	4
Proteins	9.9g	13
Total fat	35g	64
Saturated fat	19g	86
Trans fats	-	**
Dietary fiber	4.5g	18
Sodium	3.7 mg	-

* % Daily Reference Values based on a 2000 kcal or 8400 kJ diet. Your daily values may be higher or lower depending on your energy needs.
** DV not established.

Paçoquinha
Yield: 10 servings
Preparation time: 10 minutes

Ingredients

- 200g of peanuts (preferably roasted, shelled and unsalted)
- 1 cup of erythritol sweetener (or ¾ cup xylitol sweetener)
- ¼ cup of coconut flour (or almond flour)
- 50g of dried coconut flakes or chips
- 3 tablespoons of coconut oil (or softened unsalted butter)
- 1 pinch of salt

Preparation method

In a food processor, grind the peanuts and coconut into a paste. After 3 minutes, pause the processor, open it to clean the edges not picked up by the blades, and start blending again. Add the coconut oil, erythritol, and salt. Beat until it is homogeneous. Shape the dough into squares, place it in the desired shape, or place it on a tray and put it in the fridge for about 30 minutes.

| NUTRITIONAL INFORMATION ||||
| 25g serving (1 unit) ||||
	Amount per serving	%DV(*)
Energetic value	134kcal or 549kJ	7
Carbohydrates	9.7g	3
Proteins	3.0g	4
Total fat	9.2g	17
Saturated fat	4.8g	22
Trans fats	-	**
Dietary fiber	0.8g	3
Sodium	9.3 mg	-

* % Daily Reference Values based on a 2000 kcal or 8400 kJ diet. Your daily values may be higher or lower depending on your energy needs.
** DV not established.

Coconut Mousse

Yield: 4 servings

Preparation time: 1 hour and 15 minutes

Ingredients

- 1 glass of coconut milk
- 200 g dehydrated, unsweetened grated coconut
- 1 small box of cream
- 30 drops of sweetener
- 1 dessert spoon of vanilla (optional)
- ½ packet of powdered gelatin
- 1 cup of water

Preparation method

Leave the shredded coconut to hydrate for 30 minutes in the coconut milk, already sweetened with 30 drops of sweetener.

Then, add the cream, vanilla, and gelatine dissolved in 1 cup of water.

Refrigerate and consume once it is firm.

NUTRITIONAL INFORMATION			
20g serving (1 tablespoon)			
	Amount per serving		%DV(*)
Energetic value	80kcal or 336kJ		4
Carbohydrates	1.9g		1
Proteins	0.51g		1
Total fat	7.8g		14
Saturated fat	6		27
Trans fats	-		**
Dietary fiber	0.15		1
Sodium	7.7 mg		-
* % Daily Reference Values based on a 2000 kcal or 8400 kJ diet. Your daily values may be higher or lower depending on your energy needs. ** DV not established.			

Fit Truffle

Yield: 3 servings
Preparation time: 15 minutes

Ingredients

- 1 tablespoon of sugar-free peanut butter
- 1 tablespoon of oat bran
- 1 tablespoon of xylitol sweetener
- 1 tablespoon of cocoa powder

Preparation method

All you have to do is mix all the ingredients and stir until it becomes a homogeneous mixture. Then, just make balls and dip them in cocoa.

NUTRITIONAL INFORMATION		
25g serving (1 unit)		
	Amount per serving	%DV(*)
Energetic Value	84kcal or 344kJ	4
Carbohydrates	9.9g	3
Proteins	4.1g	5
Total fat	3.1g	6
Saturated fat	0.7g	3
Trans fats	-	**
Dietary fiber	3.4g	14
Sodium	2.2 mg	-
* % Daily Reference Values based on a 2000 kcal or 8400 kJ diet. Your daily values may be higher or lower depending on your energy needs. ** DV not established.		

Low Carb Biscuit

Yield: 15 servings
Preparation time: 35 minutes

Ingredients

- 1 cup of cashew nuts
- 1 + ½ cup of coconut flour
- 1/3 cup of coconut milk
- 1/3 cup of dark chocolate chips
- 3 tablespoons of xylitol
- 1 teaspoon of baking soda

Preparation method

Blend the cashew nuts until they turn into flour, then pour into a bowl. Add the other ingredients (except chocolate) and mix well. Mold the cookies, place them in a mold, and put the chocolate drops on top. Bake for approximately 15 minutes over medium heat.

NUTRITIONAL INFORMATION 30g serving (1 unit)		
	Amount per serving	%DV(*)
Energetic value	105kcal or 430kJ	5
Carbohydrates	6.5g	2
Proteins	2.1g	3
Total fat	7.9g	14
Saturated fat	2.9g	13
Trans fats	-	**
Dietary fiber	1.0g	4
Sodium	90 mg	4

* % Daily Reference Values based on a 2000 kcal or 8400 kJ diet. Your daily values may be higher or lower depending on your energy needs.
** DV not established.

Spoon Cocada
Yield: 9 servings

Preparation time: 60 minutes

Ingredients

- 2 cups of grated dry coconut
- 2 tablespoons of xylitol
- 1 cup of skimmed milk powder
- 1 cup of milk and
- 1 tablespoon of cornstarch

Preparation method

Place the coconut in a non-stick or greased pan and set aside. In a blender, beat the milk, sugar, powdered milk, and starch. Once blended, cook over low heat, stirring until it thickens. Pour over the grated coconut and bake in a medium oven for about 40 minutes until the milk thickens and turns yellow. The texture is soft, so that you can eat it with a spoon.

\multicolumn{3}{c	}{NUTRITIONAL INFORMATION}
\multicolumn{3}{c	}{20g serving (1 tablespoon)}
	Amount per serving	%DV(*)
Energetic value	95kcal or 389kJ	5
Carbohydrates	6.0g	2
Proteins	2.4g	3
Total fat	6.8g	12
Saturated fat	5.8g	26
Trans fats	-	**
Dietary fiber	-	-
Sodium	36 mg	1

* % Daily Reference Values based on a 2000 kcal or 8400 kJ diet. Your daily values may be higher or lower depending on your energy needs.
** DV not established.

Fruit Salad with Ricotta and Yogurt
Yield: 800g
Preparation time: 45 minutes

Ingredients

- 250g of fresh ricotta
- 400 grams of Greek yogurt
- ½ cup of coconut milk
- 4 tablespoons of culinary sweetener
- 1 teaspoon of vanilla extract
- 1 chopped kiwi
- chopped strawberries
- 1 chopped mango

Preparation method

Place the coconut milk, yogurt, vanilla, sweetener, and ricotta in a blender. Blend until smooth, about 5 minutes.

Place in the freezer for 30 minutes until it gains more consistency. Assemble in individual cups, mixing the cream with the chopped fruit.

NUTRITIONAL INFORMATION 75g serving (1 cup)		
	Amount per serving	%DV(*)
Energetic value	70kcal or 294kJ	3
Carbohydrates	9.6g	3
Proteins	5g	7
Total fat	5.2g	9
Saturated fat	3.4g	15
Trans fats	-	**
Dietary fiber	0.45g	2
Sodium	108 mg	4

* % Daily Reference Values based on a 2000 kcal or 8400 kJ diet. Your daily values may be higher or lower depending on your energy needs.
** DV not established.

Blueberry detox

Ingredients

- 200 ml of water
- 5 spinach leaves
- ½ frozen banana
- ½ cup of blueberries (blueberries)

Preparation method

Blend everything in the blender. Serve chilled.

NUTRITIONAL INFORMATION 200ml serving (1 glass)		
	Amount per serving	%DV(*)
Energetic value	83kcal or 349kJ	4
Carbohydrates	19g	6
Proteins	1.7g	2
Total fat	-	-
Saturated fat	-	-
Trans fats	-	**
Dietary fiber	2.8g	11
Sodium	18 mg	1

* % Daily Reference Values based on a 2000 kcal or 8400 kJ diet. Your daily values may be higher or lower depending on your energy needs.
** DV not established.

Lemon Smoothie with Coconut Milk

Ingredients

- Lemon juice (½ medium lemon)
- 3 tablespoons of coconut milk
- 2 tablespoons of xylitol
- Mint leaves to taste
- Ice to taste

Preparation method

Blend all ingredients in a blender until foamy.

NUTRITIONAL INFORMATION		
200ml serving (1 glass)		
	Amount per serving	%DV(*)
Energetic value	171kcal or 701kJ	8
Carbohydrates	19g	6
Proteins	1.2g	2
Total fat	10g	18
Saturated fat	9.5g	43
Trans fats	-	**
Dietary fiber	1.2g	5
Sodium	6.7 mg	-

* % Daily Reference Values based on a 2000 kcal or 8400 kJ diet. Your daily values may be higher or lower depending on your energy needs.
** DV not established.

Strawberry Ice Cream

Yield: 3 servings

Preparation time: 10 minutes

Ingredients

- 1 cup of (200 ml) coconut milk or cream (leave in the fridge overnight)
- 3 cups of frozen strawberries

Preparation method

Mix in a blender or food processor until desired consistency is achieved. It can be served with strawberries and coconut shavings.

| NUTRITIONAL INFORMATION |||
| 60g serving (1 scoop of ice cream) |||
	Amount per serving	%DV(*)
Energetic value	53kcal or 217kJ	3
Carbohydrates	3.1g	1
Proteins	0.6g	1
Total fat	4.2g	8
Saturated fat	3.7g	17
Trans fats	-	**
Dietary fiber	0.8g	3
Sodium	2.8 mg	-

* % Daily Reference Values based on a 2000 kcal or 8400 kJ diet. Your daily values may be higher or lower depending on your energy needs.
** DV not established.

Cream Ice Cream

Yield: 20 servings
Preparation time: 5 minutes

Ingredients

- 200 g (1 cup) of cream
- 200g (1 cup) of cream
- 90g (1/2 cup) of erythritol
- 15g of coconut oil
- Vanilla essence
- ½ cc of xanthan gum or agar agar

Preparation method

Blend the ingredients in a blender or a mixer until you obtain a homogeneous mixture. Place the mixture in an ice cream machine, following the manufacturer's instructions. Place the mixture in the freezer for 4 hours, stirring every 30 minutes.

Then, let it rest in the freezer for another 2 to 4 hours.

| NUTRITIONAL INFORMATION |||
| 60g serving (1 scoop of ice cream) |||
	Amount per serving	%DV(*)
Energetic value	153kcal or 627kJ	8
Carbohydrates	1.4g	-
Proteins	0.9g	1
Total fat	16g	29
Saturated fat	12g	54
Trans fats	-	**
Dietary fiber	0.5g	2
Sodium	11 mg	-

* % Daily Reference Values based on a 2000 kcal or 8400 kJ diet. Your daily values may be higher or lower depending on your energy needs.
** DV not established.

Final message

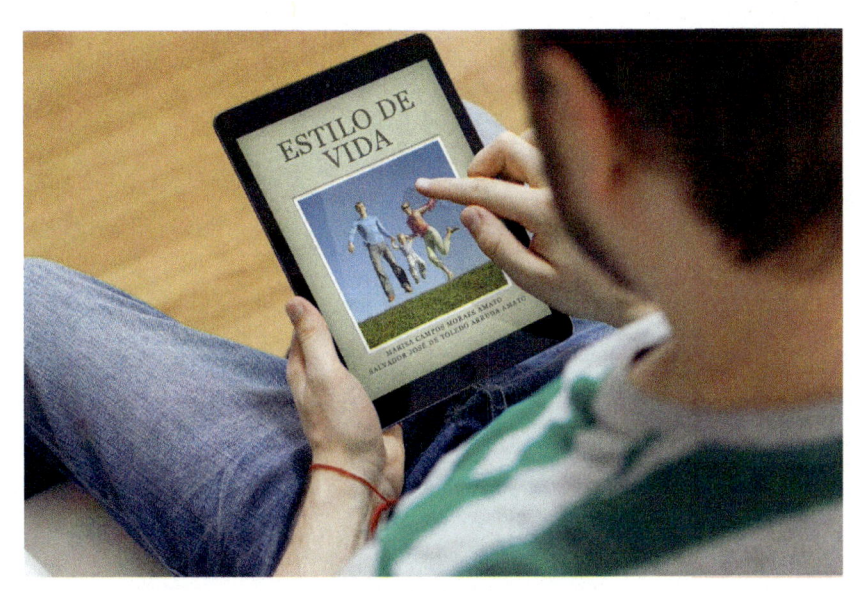

You, who have come this far, deserve a treat!

Therefore, I am giving you the book **Estilo de Vida** for iOS, which can be downloaded here at this link: https://bio.amato.io/estilo

I just ask that you comment, rate this book, and tell us how you acquired it at https://bio.amato.io/cetogenica

I need testimonials to spread this message and help more people.

Share it with your friends and colleagues, post it on your social media, and help spread the word about the benefits of the ketogenic diet.

I would also like to see you on our YouTube channel: https://bio.amato.io/youtube or, perhaps, on Instagram: https://bio.amato.io/insta-ale, where my positive and constructive messages are attracting a lot of people — unlike Twitter: https://bio.amato.io/twitter-ale, whose platform I still don't understand, as it seems that only those who spread hate end up growing.

Anyway, see you on my networks!

Bibliography

1. Freeman JM, Kossoff EH, Hartman AL. The ketogenic diet: One decade later. *Pediatrics* 2007; 119: 535–543.
2. Bailey EE, Pfeifer HH, Thiele EA. The use of diet in the treatment of epilepsy. *Epilepsy Behav* 2005; 6: 4–8.
3. Broom GM, Shaw IC, Rucklidge JJ. The ketogenic diet as a potential treatment and prevention strategy for Alzheimer's disease. *Nutrition* 2019; 60: 118–121.
4. Keith L, Seo CA, Rowsemitt C, et al. Ketogenic diet as a potential intervention for lipedema. *Med Hypotheses* 2021; 146: 110435.
5. Moriconi E, Camajani E, Fabbri A, et al. Very-Low-Calorie Ketogenic Diet as a Safe and Valuable Tool for Long-Term Glycemic Management in Patients with Obesity and Type 2 Diabetes. *Nutrients* 2021; 13: 758.
6. Allen BG, Bhatia SK, Anderson CM, et al. Ketogenic diets as an adjuvant cancer therapy: History and potential mechanism. *Redox Biol* 2014; 2: 963–970.
7. Weber DD, Aminazdeh-Gohari S, Kofler B. Ketogenic diet in cancer therapy. *Aging (Albany NY)* 2018; 10: 164–165.
8. Weber DD, Aminzadeh-Gohari S, Tulipan J, et al. Ketogenic diet in the treatment of cancer – Where do we stand? *Mol Metab* 2020; 33: 102–121.
9. Napoli E, Dueñas N, Giulivi C. Potential therapeutic use of the ketogenic diet in autism spectrum disorders. *Front Pediatr* 2014; 2: 1–9.
10. Ruskin DN, Svedova J, Cote JL, et al. Ketogenic Diet Improves Core Symptoms of Autism in BTBR Mice. *PLoS One* 2013; 8: 4–9.
11. Włodarek D. Role of ketogenic diets in neurodegenerative diseases (Alzheimer's disease and parkinson's disease). *Nutrients*; 11. Epub ahead of print 2019. DOI: 10.3390/nu11010169.

12. Phillips MCL, Murtagh DKJ, Gilbertson LJ, et al. Low-fat versus ketogenic diet in Parkinson's disease: A pilot randomized controlled trial. *Mov Disord* 2018; 33: 1306–1314.
13. Di Lorenzo C, Ballerini G, Barbanti P, et al. Applications of ketogenic diets in patients with headache: Clinical recommendations. *Nutrients*; 13. Epub ahead of print 2021. DOI: 10.3390/nu13072307.
14. Maggioni F, Margoni M, Zanchin G. Ketogenic diet in migraine treatment: A brief but ancient history. *Cephalalgia* 2011; 31: 1150–1151.
15. García-Caballero M, Zecchin A, Souffreau J, et al. Role and therapeutic potential of dietary ketone bodies in lymph vessel growth. *Nat Metab* 2019; 1: 666–675.
16. Storoni M, Plant GT. The Therapeutic Potential of the Ketogenic Diet in Treating Progressive Multiple Sclerosis. *Mult Scler Int* 2015; 2015: 1–9.
17. Paoli A, Rubini A, Volek JS, et al. Beyond weight loss: A review of the therapeutic uses of very-low-carbohydrate (ketogenic) diets. *Eur J Clin Nutr* 2013; 67: 789–796.
18. Ludwig DS. The Ketogenic Diet: Evidence for Optimism but High-Quality Research Needed. *J Nutr* 2020; 150: 1354–1359.
19. Bahr LS, Bock M, Liebscher D, et al. Ketogenic diet and fasting diet as Nutritional Approaches in Multiple Sclerosis (NAMS): protocol of a randomized controlled study. 2019; 1–9.
20. Hemingway C, Freeman JM, Pillas DJ, et al. The ketogenic diet: A 3- to 6-year follow-up of 150 children enrolled prospectively. *Pediatrics* 2001; 108: 898–905.
21. Vining EPG, Freeman JM, Ballaban-Gil K, et al. A multicenter study of the efficacy of the ketogenic diet. *Arch Neurol* 1998; 55: 1433–1437.
22. Lennerz B, Lennerz JK. Food Addiction, High-Glycemic-Index Carbohydrates, and Obesity. *Clin Chem* 2018; 64: 64–71.

23. Ibrahim KS, El-Sayed EM. Dietary conjugated linoleic acid and medium-chain triglycerides for obesity management. *J Biosci*; 46. Epub ahead of print 2021. DOI: 10.1007/s12038-020-00133-3.
24. Kossoff EH, Krauss GL, McGrogan JR, et al. Efficacy of the Atkins diet as therapy for intractable epilepsy. *Neurology* 2003; 61: 1789–1791.
25. Kossoff EH, Cervenka MC, Henry BJ, et al. A decade of the modified Atkins diet (2003-2013): Results, insights, and future directions. *Epilepsy Behav* 2013; 29: 437–442.
26. de Cabo R, Mattson MP. Effects of Intermittent Fasting on Health, Aging, and Disease. *N Engl J Med* 2019; 381: 2541–2551.
27. Stewart WK, Fleming LW. Features of a successful therapeutic fast of 382 days' duration. *Postgrad Med J* 1973; 49: 203–209.
28. Wyka J, Malczyk E, Misiarz M, et al. Assessment of food intakes for women adopting the high protein Dukan diet. *Rocz Państwowego Zakładu Hig* 2015; 66: 137–142.
29. Dashti HM, Mathew TC, Khadada M, et al. Beneficial effects of ketogenic diet in obese diabetic subjects. *Mol Cell Biochem* 2007; 302: 249–256.
30. Sharman MJ, Gómez AL, Kraemer WJ, et al. Very Low-Carbohydrate and Low-Fat Diets Affect Fasting Lipids and Postprandial Lipemia Differently in Overweight Men. *J Nutr* 2004; 134: 880–885.
31. Johnstone AM, Horgan GW, Murison SD, et al. Effects of a high-protein ketogenic diet on hunger, appetite, and weight loss in obese men feeding ad libitum. *Am J Clin Nutr* 2008; 87: 44–55.
32. Salas Noain J, Minupuri A, Kulkarni A, et al. Significant Impact of the Ketogenic Diet on Low-Density Lipoprotein Cholesterol Levels. *Cureus* 2020; 12: 10–13.
33. Kephart W, Pledge C, Roberson P, et al. The Three-Month Effects of a Ketogenic Diet on Body Composition, Blood Parameters, and Performance Metrics in CrossFit Trainees: A

Pilot Study. *Sports* 2018; 6: 1.
34. Bergqvist AGC. Long-term monitoring of the ketogenic diet: Do's and Don'ts. *Epilepsy Res* 2012; 100: 261–266.
35. Dahlin M, Hjelte L, Nilsson S, et al. Plasma phospholipid fatty acids are influenced by a ketogenic diet enriched with n-3 fatty acids in children with epilepsy. *Epilepsy Res* 2007; 73: 199–207.
36. Fenton C, Chee CM, Bergqvist AGC. Manipulation of Types of Fats and Cholesterol Intake Can Successfully Improve the Lipid Profile While Maintaining the Efficacy of the Ketogenic Diet. *ICAN Infant, Child, Adolesc Nutr* 2009; 1: 338–341.
37. Sampath A, Kossoff EH, Furth SL, et al. Kidney stones and the ketogenic diet: Risk factors and prevention. *J Child Neurol* 2007; 22: 375–378.
38. Groesbeck DK, Bluml RM, Kossoff EH. Long-term use of the ketogenic diet in the treatment of epilepsy. *Dev Med Child Neurol* 2006; 48: 978–981.
39. Paoli A, Grimaldi K, D'Agostino D, et al. Ketogenic diet does not affect strength performance in elite artistic gymnasts. *J Int Soc Sports Nutr* 2012; 9: 1.
40. Wilson JM, Lowery RP, Roberts MD, et al. *Effects of Ketogenic Dieting on Body Composition, Strength, Power, and Hormonal Profiles in Resistance Training Men*. 2020. Epub ahead of print 2020. DOI: 10.1519/JSC.0000000000001935.
41. Paoli A, Grimaldi K, Bianco A, et al. Medium term effects of a ketogenic diet and a Mediterranean diet on resting energy expenditure and respiratory ratio. *BMC Proc* 2012; 6: P37.
42. DeFronzo RA, Tripathy D. Skeletal muscle insulin resistance is the primary defect in type 2 diabetes. *Diabetes Care*; 32 Suppl 2. Epub ahead of print 2009. DOI: 10.2337/dc09-s302.
43. Volek JS, Freidenreich DJ, Saenz C, et al. Metabolic characteristics of keto-adapted ultra-endurance runners. *Metabolism* 2016; 65: 100–110.
44. Zhou W, Mukherjee P, Kiebish MA, et al. The calorically restricted ketogenic diet, an effective alternative therapy for

malignant brain cancer. *Nutr Metab* 2007; 4: 1–15.
45. Nebeling LC, Miraldi F, Shurin SB, et al. Effects of a Ketogenic Diet on Tumor Metabolism and Nutritional Status in Pediatrie Oncology Patients: Two Case Reports. *J Am Coll Nutr* 1995; 14: 202–208.
46. Abdelwahab MG, Fenton KE, Preul MC, et al. The ketogenic diet is an effective adjuvant to radiation therapy for the treatment of malignant glioma. *PLoS One* 2012; 7: 1–7.
47. Schmidt M, Pfetzer N, Schwab M, et al. Start-up of the research and pilot center for polyamides in Schwarza. *Chem Fibers Int* 1999; 49: 20.
48. Eric Westman. Keto Basics for Lymphatic & Fat Disorders : End Your Carb Confusion. In: *Ketogenic Solution for Fat and Lymphatic Disorders*, https://vimeo.com/484129984 (2020).
49. Volek JS, Phinney SD, Forsythe CE, et al. Carbohydrate restriction has a more favorable impact on the metabolic syndrome than a low fat diet. *Lipids* 2009; 44: 297–309.
50. Olefsky JM, Crapo P, Reaven D. Postprandial responses plasma triglyceride to a low-fat. *Am J Clin Nutr* 1976; 29: 535–539.
51. Batch JT, Lamsal SP, Adkins M, et al. Advantages and Disadvantages of the Ketogenic Diet: A Review Article. *Cureus* 2020; 12: 10–14.
52. Santos FL, Esteves SS, da Costa Pereira A, et al. Systematic review and meta-analysis of clinical trials of the effects of low carbohydrate diets on cardiovascular risk factors. *Obes Rev* 2012; 13: 1048–1066.
53. Amato ACM, Amato FCM, Benitti DA, et al. Criação de questionário e modelo de rastreamento de lipedema. *J Vasc Bras* 2020; 19: 1–7.
54. Allen E V, Hines EA, Hines EA. Lipedema of the legs: a syndrome characterized by fat legs and orthostatic edema. *Proc Staff Meet Mayo Clin* 1940; 15: 184–187.
55. Wold L, Hines EA, Allen E V. Lipedema of the legs: a syndrome characterized by fat legs and edema. *Ann Intern Med* 1951; 34: 1243–1250.

56. Whonamedit - dictionary of medical eponyms.pdf. *Allen-Hines syndrome*, https://www.whonamedit.com/synd.cfm/2015.html.
57. Moraes IN. Cânones da beleza. *Rev Cult e Saude* 2003; 1: 25–30.
58. Fife CE, Maus EA, Carter MJ. Lipedema: a frequently misdiagnosed and misunderstood fatty deposition syndrome. *Adv Skin Wound Care* 2010; 23: 81–84.
59. Beninson J, Edelglass JW. Lipedema - the non-lymphatic masquerader. *Angiology* 1984; 35: 506–510.
60. Reich-Schupke S, Altmeyer P, Stücker M. Thick legs - not always lipedema. *J Dtsch Dermatol Ges* 2013; 11: 225–233.
61. Forner-Cordero I, Szolnoky G, Forner-Cordero A, et al. Lipedema: an overview of its clinical manifestations, diagnosis and treatment of the disproportional fatty deposition syndrome - systematic review. *Clin Obes* 2012; 2: 86–95.
62. Herpertz U. Krankheitsspektrum des lipodems an einer lymphologischen fachklinik - erscheinungsformen, mischbilder und behandlungsmoglichkeiten. *Vasomed* 1997; 9: 301–307.
63. Okhovat J-P, Alavi A. Lipedema: A Review of the Literature. *Int J Low Extrem Wounds* 2015; 14: 262–267.
64. Goodliffe JM, Ormerod JOM, Beale A, et al. An underdiagnosed cause of leg swelling. *BMJ Case Rep*; 2013. Epub ahead of print 2013. DOI: 10.1136/bcr-2013-009538.
65. Langendoen SI, Habbema L, Nijsten TEC, et al. Lipoedema: from clinical presentation to therapy. A review of the literature. *Br J Dermatol* 2009; 161: 980–986.
66. Asmussen PD, Földi M, Strößenreuther R, et al. *Földi's textbook of lymphology for physicians and lymphedema therapists*. München: Elsevier Urban & Fischer, 2012.
67. Chen S-G, Hsu S-D, Chen T-M, et al. Painful fat syndrome in a male patient. *Br J Plast Surg* 2004; 57: 282–286.
68. Fife CE, Maus EA, Carter MJ. Lipedema: a frequently misdiagnosed and misunderstood fatty deposition syndrome. *Adv Ski Wound Care* 2010; 23: 81–84.

69. Marshall M, Schwahn-Schreiber C. Prävalenz des Lipödems bei berufstätigen Frauen in Deutschland. *Phlebologie* 2011; 40: 127–134.
70. Amato ACM, Amato FCM, Amato JLS, et al. Prevalência e fatores de risco para lipedema no Brasil. *J Vasc Bras* 2022; no prelo: 1–11.
71. Child AH, Gordon KD, Sharpe P, et al. Lipedema: an inherited condition. *Am J Med Genet A* 2010; 152A: 970–976.
72. Szél E, Kemény L, Groma G, et al. Pathophysiological dilemmas of lipedema. *Med Hypotheses* 2014; 83: 599–606.
73. Buck DW, Herbst KL. Lipedema: A Relatively Common Disease with Extremely Common Misconceptions. *Plast Reconstr Surg Glob Open* 2016; 4: e1043.
74. Dayan E, Kim JN, Smith ML, et al. *Lipedema - The Disease They Call FAT: An Overview for Clinicians*. Lipedema Simplified Publications, 2017.
75. Keith L, Rowsemitt C, Richards LG. Lifestyle Modification Group for Lymphedema and Obesity Results in Significant Health Outcomes. *101177@1559827617742108.pdf*. Epub ahead of print 2017. DOI: 10.1177/1559827617742108.
76. Amato ACM. Is Lipedema a Unique Entity? *EC Clin Med Cases Reports* 2020; 2: 1–7.
77. Siems W, Grune T, Voss P, et al. Anti-fibrosclerotic effects of shock wave therapy in lipedema and cellulite. *Biofactors* 2005; 24: 275–282.
78. Wright TF, Herbst KL. A 41-year-old woman with excessive fat of the lower body since puberty with progression to swollen ankles and feet despite caloric restriction, due to lipedema and protein-calorie malnutrition: A case of stage 3 lipedema. *Am J Case Rep* 2021; 22: 1–6.
79. Faerber G. Experiences with lipedema & keto in Germany clinic/German Standard of Care (SOC). In: *Ketogenic Solution for Fat and Lymphatic Disorders*, https://vimeo.com/484129984 (2020).
80. Apkhanova T V., Sergeev VN, Krukova MM, et al. Influence of Ketogenic Diet and Nutraceutical Correction in the

Complex Treatment of Lower Limbs Lipedema. *Vestn Vosstanov Med* 2021; 20: 26–36.
81. Hoyt LT, Falconi AM. Puberty and perimenopause: Reproductive transitions and their implications for women's health. *Soc Sci Med* 2015; 132: 103–112.
82. AL-Ghadban S, Cromer W, Allen M, et al. Dilated Blood and Lymphatic Microvessels, Angiogenesis, Increased Macrophages, and Adipocyte Hypertrophy in Lipedema Thigh Skin and Fat Tissue. *J Obes* 2019; 2019: 1–10.
83. Felmerer G, Stylianaki A, Hollmén M, et al. Increased levels of VEGF-C and macrophage infiltration in lipedema patients without changes in lymphatic vascular morphology. *Sci Rep* 2020; 10: 1–10.
84. Youm YH, Nguyen KY, Grant RW, et al. The ketone metabolite β-hydroxybutyrate blocks NLRP3 inflammasome-mediated inflammatory disease. *Nat Med* 2015; 21: 263–269.
85. Lindberg UB, Crona N, Silfverstolpe, et al. Regional adipose tissue metabolism in postmenopausal women after treatment with exogenous se steroids. *Horm Metab Res* 1990; 22: 345–351.
86. Pereira RI, Casey BA, Swibas TA, et al. Timing of estradiol treatment after menopause may determine benefit or harm to insulin action. *J Clin Endocrinol Metab* 2015; 100: 4456–4462.
87. Ivandić A, Prpić-Križevac I, Sučić M, et al. Hyperinsulinemia and sex hormones in healthy premenopausal women: Relative contribution of obesity, obesity type, and duration of obesity. *Metabolism* 1998; 47: 13–19.
88. Cohen PG. Aromatase, adiposity, aging and disease. The hypogonadal-metabolic-atherogenic-disease and aging connection. *Med Hypotheses* 2001; 56: 702–708.
89. Ruskin DN, Kawamura M, Masino SA. Reduced pain and inflammation in juvenile and adult rats fed a ketogenic diet. *PLoS One* 2009; 4: 1–6.
90. Masino SA, Ruskin DN. Ketogenic diets and pain. *J Child Neurol* 2013; 28: 993–1001.

91. Cooper MA, Menta BW, Perez-Sanchez C, et al. A ketogenic diet reduces metabolic syndrome-induced allodynia and promotes peripheral nerve growth in mice. *Exp Neurol* 2018; 306: 149–157.
92. Glass LM, Dickson RC, Anderson JC, et al. Total Body Weight Loss of ≥10 % Is Associated with Improved Hepatic Fibrosis in Patients with Nonalcoholic Steatohepatitis. *Dig Dis Sci* 2015; 60: 1024–1030.
93. Tendler D, Lin S, Yancy WS, et al. The effect of a low-carbohydrate, ketogenic diet on nonalcoholic fatty liver disease: A pilot study. *Dig Dis Sci* 2007; 52: 589–593.
94. Peng Y, Rideout DA, Rakita SS, et al. Does lkb1 mediate activation of hepatic amp-protein kinase (ampk) and sirtuin1 (sirt1) after roux-en-y gastric bypass in obese rats? *J Gastrointest Surg* 2010; 14: 221–228.
95. Paoli A. Ketogenic diet for obesity: Friend or foe? *Int J Environ Res Public Health* 2014; 11: 2092–2107.
96. Carmienke S, Freitag MH, Pischon T, et al. General and abdominal obesity parameters and their combination in relation to mortality: A systematic review and meta-regression analysis. *Eur J Clin Nutr* 2013; 67: 573–585.
97. Volek JS, Sharman MJ, Gómez AL, et al. Comparison of energy-restricted very low-carbohydrate and low-fat diets on weight loss and body composition in overweight men and women. *Nutr Metab* 2004; 1: 1–13.
98. Faloia E, Tirabassi G, Canibus P, et al. Protective effect of leg fat against cardiovascular risk factors in obese premenopausal women. *Nutr Metab Cardiovasc Dis* 2009; 19: 39–44.
99. Santos RD, Gagliardi ACM, Xavier HT, et al. I diretriz sobre o consumo de gorduras e saúde cardiovascular. *Arq Bras Cardiol* 2013; 100: 1–40.
100. Izar MC de O, Lottenberg AM, Giraldez VZR, et al. Posicionamento sobre o Consumo de Gorduras e Saúde Cardiovascular – 2021. *Arq Bras Cardiol* 2021; 116: 160–212.
101. Bridge E, Iob L. The mechanism of the ketogenic diet in epilepsy. *Bull Johns Hopkins Hosp*.

102. Berryman MS. The ketogenic diet revisited. *J Am Diet Assoc* 1997; 97: 743–749.
103. Bough KJ, Rho JM. Anticonvulsant mechanisms of the ketogenic diet. *Epilepsia* 2007; 48: 43–58.
104. Bough KJ, Wetherington J, Hassel B, et al. Mitochondrial biogenesis in the anticonvulsant mechanism of the ketogenic diet. *Ann Neurol* 2006; 60: 223–235.
105. Fonseca do V, Francine P, Furian D. Diferenças Da Carne De Animais Criados Em Confinamento Ou À Pasto. 2012; 4.
106. Patterson E, Wall R, Fitzgerald GF, et al. Health implications of high dietary omega-6 polyunsaturated fatty acids. *J Nutr Metab*; 2012. Epub ahead of print 2012. DOI: 10.1155/2012/539426.
107. F DA, C G, L R. Evaluation of Chemical and Physical Changes in Different Commercial Oils during Heating. *Acta Sci Nutr Heal* 2018; 2: 02–11.
108. Zilch M, Soares B, Bennemann G, et al. Análise da ingestão de proteínas e suplementação por praticantes de musculação nas academias centrais da cidade de Guarapuava-PR. *Rev Bras Nutr Esportiva* 2012; 6: 7.
109. Menon D, Santos JS dos. CONSUMO DE PROTEÍNA POR PRATICANTES DE MUSCULAÇÃO QUE OBJETIVAM HIPERTROFIA MUSCULAR PROTEIN CONSUMPTION BY BODYBUILDING PRACTITIONERS AIMING MUSCLE HYPERTROPHY Artigo originAl CLÍNICA MÉDICA DO EXERCÍCIO E DO ESPORTE. *Rev Bras Med Esporte* 2012; 18: 8–12.
110. DOSE E DISTRIBUIÇÃO DE PROTEÍNAS PARA PRATICANTES DE ATIVIDADE FÍSICA. 2017; 210093.
111. Rezende ET, Godinho SE, Souza ACN de M, et al. Ingestão Proteica E Necessidades Nutricionais De Universitários Vegetarianos. *Rev Bras Ciên Saúde* 2015; 13: 52–57.
112. Anselmo MA de C, Burini RC, Angeleli AYO, et al. Avaliação do estado nutricional de indivíduos adultos sadios de classe média: ingestão energética e protéica, antropometria, exames bioquímicos do sangue e testes de imunocompetência.

Rev Saude Publica 1992; 26: 46–53.
113. Marchini JS, Rodrigues MMP, Cunha SFC, et al. Cálculo das recomendações de ingestão protéica: aplicação a pré-escolar, escolar e adulto utilizando alimentos brasileiros. *Rev Saude Publica* 1994; 28: 146–152.
114. Pereira-Da-Silva EM, Orsoli DN, Araújo LF, et al. Hability of protein intake regulation in nile tilapia, Oreochromis niloticus. *Rev Bras Zootec* 2004; 33: 1921–1927.
115. Crescenzi R, Marton A, Donahue PMC, et al. Tissue Sodium Content is Elevated in the Skin and Subcutaneous Adipose Tissue in Women with Lipedema. *Obesity* 2018; 26: 310–317.
116. Crescenzi R, Donahue PMC, Petersen KJ, et al. Upper and Lower Extremity Measurement of Tissue Sodium and Fat Content in Patients with Lipedema. *Obesity* 2020; 28: 907–915.

Printed in Great Britain
by Amazon